Workplace Wellness Programs Study

Final Report

Soeren Mattke, Hangsheng Liu, John P. Caloyeras, Christina Y. Huang,
Kristin R. Van Busum, Dmitry Khodyakov, Victoria Shier

RAND Health

Sponsored by the U.S. Department of Labor and the U.S. Department of Health and Human Services

The research described in this report was sponsored by the U.S. Department of Labor and the U.S. Department of Health and Human Services. The work was conducted in RAND Health, a division of the RAND Corporation.

The RAND Corporation is a nonprofit institution that helps improve policy and decisionmaking through research and analysis. RAND's publications do not necessarily reflect the opinions of its research clients and sponsors.

RAND® is a registered trademark.

© Copyright 2013 RAND Corporation

Permission is given to duplicate this document for personal use only, as long as it is unaltered and complete. Copies may not be duplicated for commercial purposes. Unauthorized posting of RAND documents to a non-RAND website is prohibited. RAND documents are protected under copyright law. For information on reprint and linking permissions, please visit the RAND permissions page (http://www.rand.org/publications/permissions.html).

Published 2013 by the RAND Corporation
1776 Main Street, P.O. Box 2138, Santa Monica, CA 90407-2138
1200 South Hayes Street, Arlington, VA 22202-5050
4570 Fifth Avenue, Suite 600, Pittsburgh, PA 15213-2665
RAND URL: http://www.rand.org/
To order RAND documents or to obtain additional information, contact
Distribution Services: Telephone: (310) 451-7002;
Fax: (310) 451-6915; Email: order@rand.org

Preface

This Research Report was sponsored by the U.S. Department of Labor and the U.S. Department of Health and Human Services. It is based on a review of the scientific and trade literature, a national survey of employers with at least 50 employees in the public and private sectors, statistical analyses of health plan claims and wellness program data from several employers, and case studies of five employers with established wellness programs. The report combines existing evidence and original analyses to document composition of wellness programs, describe national patterns of program uptake among employers, analyze the impact of wellness programs on health and cost outcomes, and investigate the use and impact of financial incentives to promote program uptake. This report will be of interest to national and state policymakers, employers and wellness program vendors, employer and employee advocacy organizations, health researchers, and others with responsibilities related to designing, implementing, participating in, and monitoring workplace wellness programs.

This research was conducted under contract #DOLJ089327414 with the Department of Labor, as part of a study of workplace wellness programs that is required by the Section 2705(m)(1) of the Public Health Service Act. The Task Order Officers for the project are Anja Decressin and Keith Bergstresser of the Employee Benefits Security Administration, Department of Labor, and Diane Pilkey of the Office of the Assistant Secretary for Planning and Evaluation, Department of Health and Human Services. We thank the Task Order Officers for their guidance and reviews of the document; however, we note that the material contained in this report is the responsibility of the research team and does not necessarily reflect the beliefs or opinions of the Task Order Officers, their respective agencies, or the federal government.

This research was conducted in RAND Health, a division of the RAND Corporation. A profile of RAND Health, abstracts of its publications, and ordering information can be found at www.rand.org/health. Comments or inquiries concerning this report should be sent to the lead author, Soeren Mattke, at Soeren_Mattke@rand.org or to his address at RAND: RAND Corporation, 20 Park Plaza, Suite 920, Boston, MA 02116.

Contents

Figures

Tables

Summary

Background

Over the last several decades, an epidemic of "lifestyle diseases" has developed in the United States: Unhealthy lifestyles, such as inactivity, poor nutrition, tobacco use, and frequent alcohol consumption, are driving up the prevalence of chronic disease, such as diabetes, heart disease, and chronic pulmonary conditions. These chronic conditions have become a major burden, as they lead to decreased quality of life, premature death and disability, and increased health care cost. Furthermore, although chronic disease was once thought to be a problem of older age groups, there is a shift toward onset during Americans' working age that adds to the economic burden, because of illness-related loss of productivity due to absence from work (absenteeism) and reduced performance while at work (presenteeism).

Out of concern about the impact of chronic disease on employee health and well-being, the cost of health care coverage, and competitiveness, employers are adopting health promotion and disease prevention strategies, commonly referred to as workplace wellness programs. Disease prevention programs aim either to prevent the onset of diseases (primary prevention) or to diagnose and treat disease at an early stage before complications occur (secondary prevention). Primary prevention addresses health-related behaviors and risk factors—for example, by encouraging a diet with lower fat and caloric content to prevent the onset of diabetes mellitus. Secondary prevention attempts to improve disease control—for example, by promoting medication adherence for patients with asthma to avoid symptom exacerbations that can lead to hospitalization. Health promotion is related to disease prevention in that it aims at fostering better health through behavior change. A broad range of benefits are offered under the label "workplace wellness," from multi-component programs to single interventions, and benefits can be offered by employers directly, through a vendor, group health plans, or a combination of both.

Workplace wellness takes advantage of employers' access to employees at an age when interventions can still change their long-term health trajectory. The Patient Protection and Affordable Care Act (Affordable Care Act) supports this trend with several provisions regarding health promotion and also mandated this study.

Study Objectives and Research Approach

This report addresses the requirements of 2705(m)(1) of the Public Health Service Act and answers the following research questions:

- What are the characteristics and prevalence of current workplace wellness programs?
- What is the evidence for program impact?
- What is the role of incentives under wellness programs?
- What are key facilitators of successful wellness programs?

The project has four data collection and analysis streams:

- a review of the scientific and trade literature to identify the prevalence of wellness programs, their key components, their use of incentives, their effectiveness, their return on investment, and best practices.
- the RAND Employer Survey, a national survey of employers with at least 50 employees in the public and private sectors, including federal and state agencies, to assess program prevalence, type of wellness programs, information on incentives, and perceived program impacts.
- statistical analyses of medical claims and wellness program data from a convenience sample of large employers in the Care Continuum Alliance (CCA) database to assess the effects of wellness programs on health and cost outcomes and the effect of incentives on program participation.
- five case studies of existing wellness programs in a diverse set of employers to enhance our understanding of the effectiveness of wellness programs by providing specific examples and experiences of individual employers and employees.

Characteristics and Prevalence of Workplace Wellness Programs

According to the RAND Employer Survey conducted for this study, approximately half of U.S. employers offer wellness promotion initiatives, and larger employers are more likely to have more complex wellness programs. Programs often include *wellness screening activities* to identify health risks and *interventions* to reduce risks and promote healthy lifestyles. Most employers (72 percent of those offering a wellness program) characterize their wellness programs as a combination of screening activities and interventions. Wellness benefits can be offered by employers or a vendor to all employees or through their group health plans to plan members.

Screening activities use Health Risk Assessments (HRAs), self-administered questionnaires on health-related behaviors (e.g., exercise patterns) and risk factors (e.g., body weight) and may include clinical screenings to collect biometric data—for instance, height, weight, blood pressure, and blood glucose levels. The RAND Employer Survey data suggest that 80 percent of employers with a wellness program screen their employees for health risks, and our case study results show that employers use results for program planning and evaluation and for directing employees to preventive interventions that address their health risks.

Preventive interventions can aim at *primary prevention* by targeting employees with risk factors for chronic disease (lifestyle management) and at *secondary prevention* by improving disease control in employees with manifest chronic conditions (disease management). As Figure S.1 shows, lifestyle management programs, which are offered by 77 percent of employers with a wellness program, target a broad range of risk factors, though nearly 80 percent offer nutrition and weight activities and 77 percent of employers offer smoking cessation programs. Similarly, all five case study employers offered some form of nutrition and weight loss intervention, such as onsite Weight Watchers group meetings, weight loss competitions, personalized phone support from health coaches, and smoking cessation activities through educational programs or telephonic counseling.

Figure S.1: Among Employers Offering a Lifestyle Management Program, Percentage Offering Specific Interventions

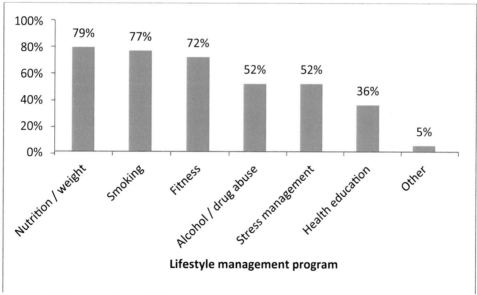

SOURCE: RAND Employer Survey, 2012.
NOTES: The graph represents information from employers with at least 50 employees that offer any lifestyle management intervention as a component of a wellness program. 51 percent of employers offer a wellness program, and 77 percent of those offer a lifestyle management intervention.

A wide variety of conditions is addressed through employer-sponsored disease management programs, as Figure S.2 depicts: Disease management programs, which 56 percent of employers with wellness programs offer, most commonly target diabetes, followed by heart disease, chronic lung disorders, depression, and cancer.

Our survey results demonstrate that, in addition to those preventive interventions, employers offer health promotion activities (86 percent), such as on-site vaccinations, healthy food options, and other health and well-being related benefits (61 percent), such as Employee Assistance Plans and on-site clinics. Case study findings suggest that employers also use population-level strategies, like health-related campaigns and wellness events.

Evidence for Program Impact

Program Uptake

Our findings suggest that uptake of worksite wellness programs remains limited. According to the RAND Employer Survey, fewer than half of employees (46 percent) undergo clinical screening and/or complete

Figure S.2: Among Employers Offering a Disease Management Program, Percentage Offering Programs for Specific Chronic Conditions

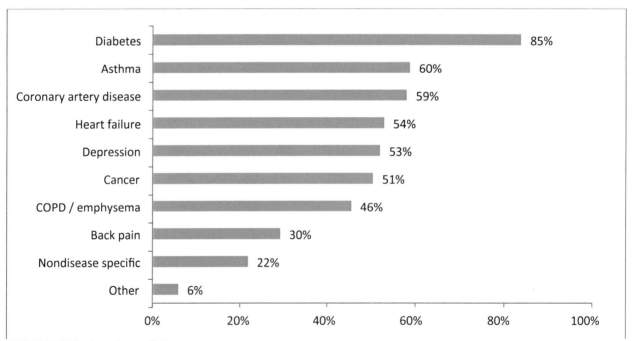

SOURCE: RAND Employer Survey, 2012.
NOTES: The graph represents information from employers with at least 50 employees that offer any disease management intervention as a component of a wellness program. 51 percent of employers offer a wellness program, and 56 percent of those offer a disease management intervention.
COPD = chronic obstructive pulmonary disease.

an HRA, which are typically used to identify employees for interventions. Of those identified for an intervention based on screening results (for example, employees who report physical activity below their recommended level), a fifth or less chose to participate, as Figure S.3 summarizes.

Program Impact on Health-Related Behaviors and Health Status

In an analysis of the CCA database, when comparing wellness program participants to statistically matched nonparticipants, we find statistically significant and clinically meaningful improvements in exercise frequency, smoking behavior, and weight control, but not cholesterol control. Those improvements are sustainable over an observation period of four years, and our simulation analyses point to cumulative effects with ongoing program participation. However, we caution that our analyses cannot account for unobservable differences between program participants and nonparticipants, such as differential motivation to change behavior.

Figure S.3: Average Participation Rates of Employees Identified for Inclusion in Select Wellness Program Components

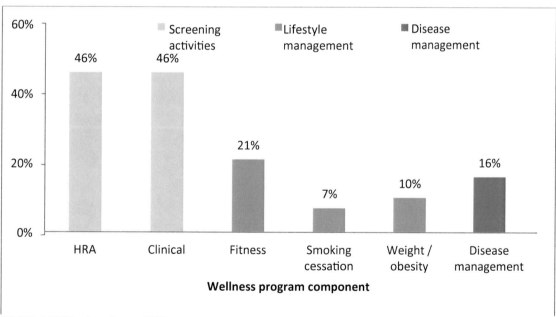

SOURCE: RAND Employer Survey, 2012.
NOTES: The graph represents information from employers with at least 50 employees that offer the specific component as part of a wellness program.
51 percent of employers offer a wellness program; of those, 65 percent conduct an HRA, 49 percent offer clinical screenings, 55 percent have a fitness program, 59 percent have smoking cessation programs, 49 percent have weight/obesity management, and 56 percent have disease management interventions. In most cases, all employees are invited to participate in screening activities, but eligibility to participate in lifestyle and disease management interventions are based on risk factors identified through screenings and health conditions identified through medical claims data, respectively. Rates reflect employees who were determined eligible for each program component.

The results show that one year participation in a weight control program is significantly associated with a reduction of body mass index (BMI) (kg/m^2) of about 0.15 in the same year, and the effect persists for two subsequent years. As illustrated in Figure S.4, this change in the first three years corresponds to a weight loss of about 0.9 pound in an average woman of 165 pounds and five feet four inches in height, or about one pound in an average man of 195 pounds and five feet nine inches in height.

The published literature, the results presented here, and our case studies corroborate the finding of positive effects of worksite wellness programs on health-related behavior and health risks among program participants. For example, a systematic review found that workplace interventions promoting smoking cessation, such as group and individual counseling and nicotine replacement therapy, increased smoking cessation rates compared to the control group. Other studies showed improvements in physical activity, higher fruit and vegetable consumption, and lower fat intake as well as a reduction in body weight, cholesterol levels, and blood pressure. One case study employer determined that roughly half of wellness program participants reported positive changes in their walking activities and eating habits, and a quarter of participants reported getting closer to a healthy weight.

Figure S.4: Effect of One-Year Participation in a Weight Control Program on Body Weight in an Average Person

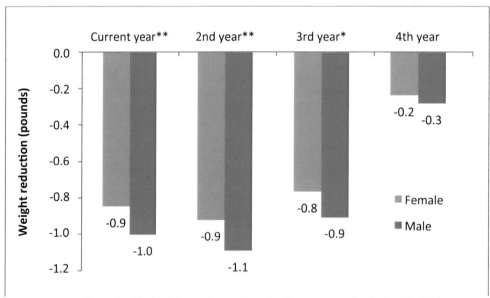

SOURCE: RAND analysis of health plan claims and screening and wellness program data in the CCA database, including 2005–2010 data from four employers and 3,924 propensity score matched pairs.
NOTES: The effects of program participation were translated to body weight reductions based on an average adult in the United States. According to the Centers for Disease Control (CDC, 2012a), the average adult female is 63.8 inches tall and weighs 164.7 pounds; the corresponding numbers for an adult male are 69.4 inches and 194.7 pounds.
*p < 0.05; **p < 0.01.

Health Care Cost and Utilization

In the RAND Employer Survey, employers overwhelmingly expressed confidence that workplace wellness programs reduce medical cost, absenteeism, and health-related productivity losses. But at the same time, only about half stated that they have evaluated program impacts formally and only 2 percent reported actual savings estimates. Similarly, none of our five case study employers had conducted a formal evaluation of their programs on cost; only one employer had requested an assessment of cost trends from its health plan. Our statistical analyses suggest that participation in a wellness program over five years is associated with a trend toward lower health care costs and decreasing health care use. We estimate the average annual difference to be $157, but the change is not statistically significant (Figure S.5).[1]

Figure S.5: Estimated Cumulative Effect of Wellness Program Participation on Total Monthly Medical Costs

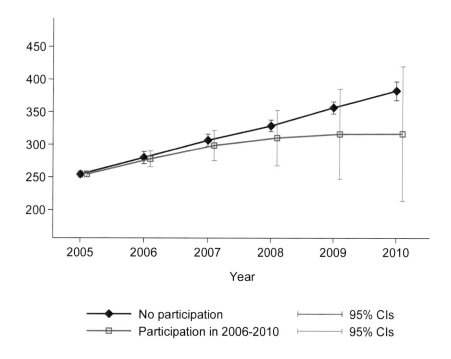

SOURCE: RAND analysis of health plan claims and screening and wellness program data in the CCA database.
NOTES: Simulation results are based on continuous participation in 2006–2010 of a population with the average characteristics of the estimation sample; p > 0.05 for all years in 2006–2010. CL = confidence interval.

---

[1] Our sample size implies that the study was adequately powered to detect an average annual change in health care cost of $378, which is well within the range of previously published estimates.

Role of Incentives in Workplace Wellness Programs

Regulations on the Use of Incentives in Workplace Wellness Programs

A number of laws and regulations at the federal and state level impose requirements and regulate the use of financial incentives in certain types of wellness programs. With respect to certain employment-based wellness programs requiring that individuals satisfy health-related standards, the Health Insurance Portability and Accountability Act (HIPAA) and the Affordable Care Act, among other things, limit incentives and require the availability of a reasonable alternative standard for certain wellness programs if for an individual it is medically inadvisable to, or it is unreasonably difficult to, achieve the standard. The Affordable Care Act raises the permissible limit on incentives for achieving a health-related standard from the prior limit of 20 percent of the cost of coverage to 30 percent in 2014. In addition, final rules being contemporaneously published at the time of this report[2] allow employers with wellness programs designed to prevent or reduce tobacco use to charge tobacco users up to 50 percent more in premiums than nonusers (*Federal Register*, 2012).

Incentives may be provided in various forms, such as premium discounts, waivers of cost-sharing requirements, or improved benefits. However, incentives that require employees to meet a health-related standard, such as target body weight, may not exceed these limits when administered by an employer's group health plan, irrespective of whether the incentives take the form of a reward, a penalty, or a combination of both. Incentives that are not tied to a health-related standard, such as participation in a diagnostic testing program, are not held to these incentive limits, so long as the incentive is available to all similarly situated individuals, and comply with other applicable federal laws, such as the Genetic Information and Nondiscrimination Act (GINA) and the Americans with Disabilities Act (ADA), and state laws.

Overall Use and Administration of Incentives

The RAND Employer Survey results indicate that nationally, more than two-thirds of employers (69 percent) with at least 50 employees and workplace wellness programs use financial incentives to encourage program uptake, and 10 percent use incentives that are tied to health-related standards.

---

[2] The Departments of Health and Human Services, Labor, and the Treasury issued a Notice for Proposed Rulemaking regarding incentives for nondiscriminatory wellness programs in group health plans on November 26, 2012 (*Federal Register*, 2012). Final rules regarding incentives for nondiscriminatory wellness programs in group health plans are being contemporaneously published with this report (*Federal Register*, 2013).

About half of employers (49 percent) with wellness programs offer incentives directly to all employees,[3] whereas 31 percent administer them through their group health plans. A fifth of employers (20 percent) administer incentives both directly and through their plans. Larger employers are more likely than smaller employers to administer their incentive schemes themselves.

We also find that results-based incentives are more commonly administered by the employer directly rather than through the health plan and linked to health coverage. According to the RAND Employer Survey, about 7 percent of employers that offer wellness programs reported administering results-based incentives through their health plans (Figure S.6). The average amount of results-based incentives for these employers was less than 10 percent of the total cost of health coverage, far from the current regulatory threshold.

Incentives for Participation in Screenings and Interventions

According to the RAND Employer Survey, the most common types of incentive triggers are HRA completion and participation in lifestyle management interventions; each is offered by about 30 percent of employers with a wellness program.

Incentives are typically framed as rewards, with 84 percent of employers reportedly using rewards rather than penalties. Incentives are offered in financial form (e.g., cash or health insurance premium surcharges) and novelty items (e.g., t-shirts or gift cards). Novelty items were used by nearly half of all employers who offer any incentives. Gym discounts (42 percent) and cash incentives (21 percent) were cited as common ways to reward program participants and/or health-related behaviors. Four out of five employers in our case studies reported using some form of financial incentive, and all five employers used novelties (e.g., t-shirts, tickets to events, and coffee mugs) as a strategy to engage employees (see Table S.1)

---

[3] HIPAA, wellness program rules, and the Affordable Care Act wellness program provisions relating to incentives for nondiscriminatory wellness programs apply with respect to incentives offered through both self-funded and insured group health plan coverage. Although Incentives that are not offered through group health plan coverage would not be subject to these requirements, other nondiscrimination and privacy laws may still apply with respect to employer practices relating to wellness programs operated outside the group health plan context.

Figure S.6: Percentage of Employers with Wellness Programs Using Participation and Results-Based Incentives for Selected Health Behaviors

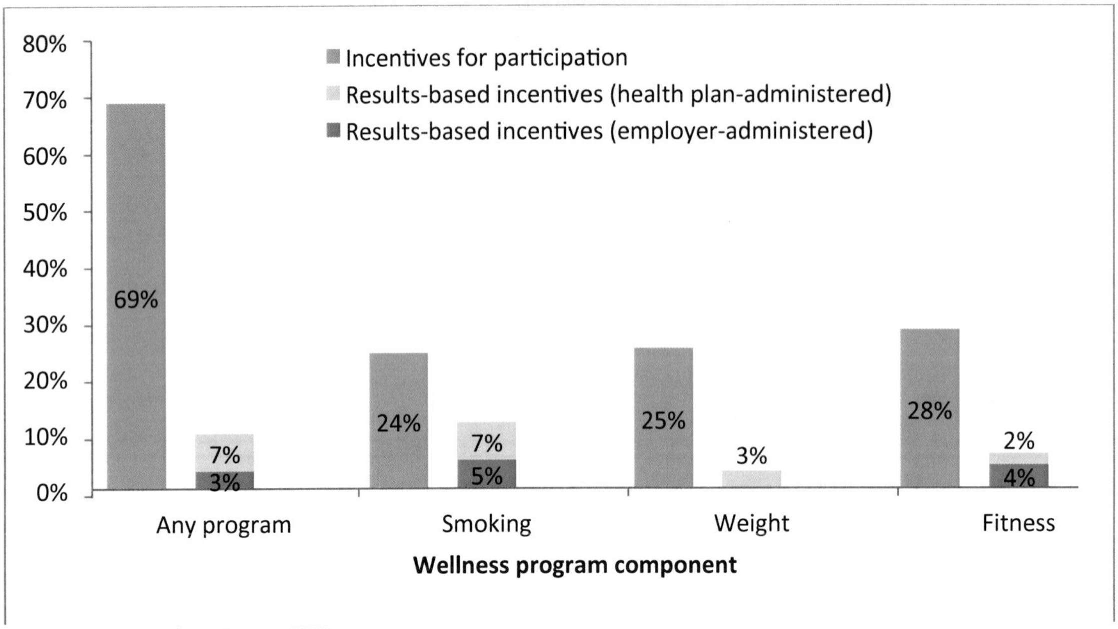

SOURCE: RAND Employer Survey, 2012.
NOTES: The graph represents information from employers with at least 50 employees with wellness programs or which offer lifestyle management as a component of a wellness program. 51 percent of employers offer a wellness program, and 77 percent of those have lifestyle management. Among employers with a lifestyle management intervention, 77 percent offer programs that target smoking, 79 percent target weight management, and 72 percent offer fitness programs.

According to the RAND Employer Survey, employers use incentives to increase employee participation in wellness screening activities (31 percent for HRA completion and 20 percent for clinical screenings) and encourage employees to join intervention programs (30 percent for lifestyle management and 4 percent for disease management). Employers who use incentives for screening activities report significantly higher participation rates than those who do not (63 percent versus 29 percent for HRA completion and 57 percent versus 38 percent for clinical screenings).

Table S.1: Percentage of Employers That Offer Monetary Incentives to Encourage Participation in Wellness Activities

Type of Component	% of All Employers That Offer a Wellness Program	% of All Employers
HRA completion	31	16
Clinical screening	20	10
Lifestyle management	30	15
Disease management	4	2
At least one component	69	35

SOURCE: RAND Employer Survey, 2012.
NOTE: The table represents the subset of employers with at least 50 employees that offer a wellness program (51 percent).

Analysis of the CCA data indicates that incentives for HRA completion are effective, particularly above a threshold of $50. Using a simulation model, we find that the incentive amount for HRA completion had a significant effect on HRA completion rates. On average, we estimate that an increase in the HRA incentive by $10 is associated with a 1.6 percentage point increase in the HRA completion rate for incentives in the range of $0–$100.

Incentives for Changes in Behavior and Health Standards

Data from the RAND Employer Survey indicate that smoking cessation is the behavior that is primarily targeted with incentives tied to health standards.[4] About a fifth of employers with smoking cessation programs (19 percent) reward actual smoking cessation, almost as many as those that reward program participation (21 percent). For other behaviors (e.g., diet), in contrast, employers were three to four times more likely to reward participation in programs than behavior change or outcomes.

Smoking is also the only health risk behavior for which achieving the goal is rewarded with a higher incentive than participation in a program. According to the RAND Employer Survey, the average incentive ($682, or 12.6% of cost of insurance coverage[5]) paid for stopping tobacco use is more than triple the incentive paid for program participation ($203). Similarly, four out of five case study employers penalized smokers, but only two had incentives tied to other health standards. The peer-reviewed literature indicates that financial incentives may attract individuals to enroll or participate in smoking cessation programs and increase initial quit rates, but they generally do not achieve long-term behavior change (Cahill and Perera, 2011; Osilla et al., 2012). Results from one randomized control trial found that large incentives (of up to $750 over the course of a year) were effective in improving abstinence rates, even when incentives were no longer offered (Volpp et al., 2009).

With respect to effectiveness, our analyses of employer data in the CCA database imply that incentives for HRA completion and program participation can significantly reduce weight and smoking rates and increase exercise. However the size of these effects is small and unlikely to be clinically meaningful.[6]

---

[4] To reduce the burden on respondents, the survey did not ask employers to specify in detail whether incentives are offered under their group health plans.

[5] According to KFF/HRET (2011), "The average premium for single coverage in 2011 is $452 per month or $5,429 per year." (KFF/HRET, 2011)

[6] Based on the Framingham Heart Study general cardiovascular disease risk model (http://www.framinghamheartstudy.org/risk/gencardio_bmi.xls) , the effects of an incentive of $100 on BMI and smoking

Key Facilitators of Successful Wellness Programs

Five factors to promote wellness program success emerged from our case study analysis and the
literature review:

- **Effective communication strategies:** All five organizations in our case studies employ strategies
  to communicate wellness program information to employees, ranging from face-to-face
  interaction to mass dissemination. Employers cited the importance of broad outreach and clear
  messaging from organizational leaders, especially for those organizations with a large and
  geographically dispersed workforce.

**Figure S.7: Average Incentive Amounts to Target Select Health Behaviors among
Employers Offering Incentives**

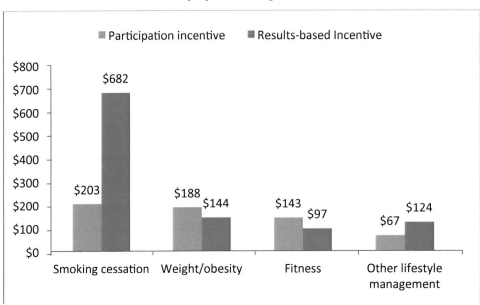

SOURCE: RAND Employer Survey, 2012.
NOTES: The graph represents information from employers with at least 50 employees that offer a monetary
incentive for participation in a lifestyle management intervention or for improving health behaviors. 51 percent
of employers offer a wellness program, and 77 percent of those include a lifestyle management intervention.
Among employers with lifestyle management interventions, 77 percent target smoking, 79 percent target
weight and obesity, and 72 percent target fitness.

- **Opportunity for employees to engage:** Those included in the case study discussions revealed
  that making wellness activities convenient and easily accessible for all employees are strategies
  that employers use to raise the level of employee engagement. Some focus group participants
  cited limited access to wellness benefits because of wait times and rigid work schedules.

---

translate to an avoidance of 11.5 cases cardiovascular disease per 10,000 population in male and 2.3 cases in female, over a
ten-year period.

- **Leadership engaged at all levels:** Evidence from case studies suggests that for programs to be a success, senior managers need to consider wellness an organizational priority to shift the company culture. Buy-in from direct supervisors is crucial to generate excitement and connect employees to available resources.
- **Use of existing resources and relationships:** All organizations in our case studies leverage existing resources and build relationships, often with health plans, to expand offerings at little to no cost.
- **Continuous evaluation:** Organizations from our case studies approach wellness with a continuous quality improvement attitude. Though no employers from our case studies conducted formal evaluations, all five solicit feedback from staff with the goal of improving future wellness programming. Three employers conducted needs assessments to develop an understanding of the wellness needs of their workforce.

Conclusions

This project represents the most comprehensive analysis of worksite wellness programs to date and evaluates current program participation, program effects, and the role of incentives. Our project combined a literature review, a national survey of employers, case studies of workplace wellness programs, and statistical analyses of medical claims and program data to assess the current use of workplace wellness programs in the United States, to estimate the effect of programs on employee health and health care cost, and to evaluate the role of incentives in program engagement.

Characteristics and Prevalence of Workplace Wellness Programs

We find that that workplace wellness programs have emerged as a common employer-sponsored benefit that is now available at about half of U.S. employers with 50 or more employees, a group that employs three-quarters of the U.S. workforce. Large employers are more likely than small employees to offer a wellness program and also tend to offer programs with a greater variety of options. Most employers are committed to long-term support of wellness programs, regarding them as a viable strategy to contain health care costs, thereby ensuring the affordability of health coverage. In spite of their popularity among employers, the impact of wellness programs are rarely formally evaluated.

Evidence on Program Impact

Consistent with prior research, we find that lifestyle management interventions as part of workplace wellness programs can reduce risk factors, such as smoking, and increase healthy behaviors, such as exercise. We find that these effects are sustainable over time and clinically meaningful. This result is of critical importance, as it confirms that workplace wellness programs can help contain the current epidemic of lifestyle-related diseases, the main driver of premature morbidity and mortality as well as health care cost in the United States. An important question for further research is how program design and implementation can improve program effects.

Our estimates of wellness program effects on health care cost are lower than most results reported in the literature, but we caution that our approach estimated the isolated effect of lifestyle management interventions, whereas many published studies captured the effect of an employer's overall approach to health and wellness. Although we do not detect statistically significant decreases in cost and use of emergency department and hospital care, the trends in health care costs und use of high-cost care for program participants and nonparticipants diverge over time. Therefore, there is reason to believe that a reduction in direct medical costs would materialize if employees continued to participate in a wellness program. Lacking access to proprietary information on program cost, we could not estimate program effects on overall cost of coverage directly, but judging by published program cost data, the programs would be cost-neutral after five program years (Baicker, Cutler and Song, 2010).

Role of Incentives in Workplace Wellness Programs

Since limited employee engagement is regarded as an important obstacle to program success, employers are using incentives to increase employee engagement, as the RAND Employer Survey and other surveys suggest. Our statistical analyses show that incentives of over $50 appear effective in getting employees to complete an HRA. Although we cannot assess the effect of higher incentives systematically, as $100 was the maximum amount used by the employers in the CCA database, case study evidence suggests that larger incentives can be effective, such as the $50 per week that Employer D in our case studies used to achieve almost 100 percent participation in onsite clinical screenings. Modest incentives also seem to increase participation in and impact of lifestyle management programs.

The use of incentives tied to health standards remains uncommon. The RAND Employer Survey shows that nationally, only 10 percent of employers with 50 or more employees that offer a wellness program use any such incentives, and only 7 percent link the incentives to premiums for health coverage. For this subset, maximum incentive amounts average less than 10 percent of the employee premium for health care coverage. The one health risk factor for which results-based incentives are more common and involve higher amounts is smoking, as suggested by both the RAND Employer Survey and our case studies.

Limitations

We need to caution that our survey results may be subject to response bias, as some characteristics of respondents and nonrespondents differed significantly. Further, both the external and internal validity of the results based on the CCA data may be limited. The database represents a convenience sample of employers with long-standing commitment and substantial investment into wellness programs, implying that results may not be generalizable to all employers. As with any nonexperimental design, we cannot fully rule out that unobservable differences between program participants and nonparticipants have influenced our results. For example, differential motivation may have contributed to our estimated effect on health behaviors, such as exercise and smoking. Finally, the limited variation in incentive use among the employers in the CCA database prevents us from reaching definite conclusions regarding the effect of incentives on wellness program participation, health behaviors, and outcomes.

Opportunities for Future Research

This project represents the most comprehensive analysis of worksite wellness programs to date, and it evaluates current program participation, program impact, and the role of incentives. It also helps us to identify priority areas for future research:

- **Long-term impact of wellness programs.** Given the long latency between health risks and development of manifest chronic diseases, a much longer follow-up period will be required to fully capture the effect of worksite wellness programs on health outcomes and cost.
- **Design of programs.** Research is needed on program design features that are most likely to achieve wellness goals. Smoking cessation is an area where additional research could inform program development. A more granular look at different program components would provide valuable insights into the determinants of program success. For example, such analyses could compare the differential effects of modalities for program delivery (e.g., telephone, Internet, and in-person). Research into the relative impact of individual-level and workforce-level interventions could help to increase program efficiency.

- **Impact on a broad range of measures.** Future studies should look at a broader range of outcomes, in particular work-related outcomes and health-related quality of life. Work-related outcomes, such as absenteeism, productivity, and retention, are of critical importance to employers as they directly affect business performance.

- **Contextual factors that modify program impact.** Contextual factors will influence the effectiveness and cost-effectiveness of workplace wellness interventions. Employer characteristics, such as workplace culture and leadership support, might modify the effect of wellness programs. Understanding the role of such modifying factors should be considered for future research. Similarly, we need to understand better how employee demographic characteristics drive decisions about program uptake and how those factors interact with financial incentives.

- **Effect of financial incentives.** "High-powered" incentives that tie a substantial proportion of the cost of coverage to specific health standards remain rare. Thus, comprehensive evaluation of the intended and unintended effects of such incentives and different incentive amounts may require a prospective or even experimental study. In addition, there is limited information on the differential impact of different incentive types (e.g., whether rewards have a different effect from penalties and whether premium reductions have a different effect from cash payments) and of changes in incentives over time.

Acknowledgments

We would like to thank our Task Order Officers, Anja Decressin and Keith Bergstresser of the Employee Benefits Security Administration, Department of Labor, and Diane Pilkey and Wilma Robinson of the Office of the Assistant Secretary for Planning and Evaluation, Department of Health and Human Services for their guidance and review of this report.

We want to express our gratitude to the Care Continuum Alliance for providing us with the data for our analyses of program impact through its Data Aggregation Project. Particular thanks go to the project team at the Care Continuum Alliance, Jeanette May, Karen Moseley, and Sue Jennings. We also thank the other members of the Data Aggregation Project, Michael Connor, Pat Ducher, John Howard, and John Rodriguez from Alere Health; Jennifer Flynn from the Mayo Clinic; and many others who wished to remain anonymous as well as the employers who permitted us to use their data for the project.

We want to express our appreciation to program staff, experts, and focus group participants at the case study employers for hosting us and providing invaluable color and context to our analysis, to clinicians, benefits consultants, academics, and experts in the field who took the time to provide thoughtful input and valuable data to the research team; to The Kaiser Family Foundation for generously sharing the questionnaire for the 2011 Annual Survey of Employer Health Benefits, which we used as a reference in designing our employer survey; and to Mercer for providing useful findings from the 2009 National Survey of Employer-Sponsored Health Plans. In addition to those contributors, we thank a number of other individuals and organizations who participated anonymously.

Many staff members at RAND helped us to realize this project. In particular, we thank Melissa Bradley and her team from RAND's Survey Research Group, who administered the employer survey, Patrick Orr for supporting the project team and the production of the report, and Daniela Golinelli, John Adams, Q Burkhart, and Nancy Nicosia who provided input into the statistical design. The RAND Health Quality Assurance process employs peer reviewers, including at least one reviewer who is external to the RAND Corporation. This study benefited from the rigorous technical reviews of Christine Eibner at RAND and Kim Jinnett, Research Director at the Integrated Benefits Institute.

Abbreviations

ADA	Americans with Disabilities Act
BMI	body mass index
CCA	Care Continuum Alliance
CDC	Centers for Disease Control and Prevention
CL	confidence level
COBRA	Consolidated Omnibus Budget Reconciliation Act
COPD	chronic obstructive pulmonary disease
CPI	consumer price index
D&B	Dun & Bradstreet
DHHS	Department of Health and Human Services
DUNS	Data Universal Numbering System
EAP	Educational Assistance Program
ERISA	Employee Retirement Income Security Act
GINA	Genetic Information and Nondiscrimination Act
HIPAA	Health Insurance Portability and Accountability Act
HMO	health maintenance organization
HRA	Health Risk Assessment
HRET	Health Research & Educational Trust
IBI	Integrated Benefits Institute
KFF	Kaiser Family Foundation
LM	lifestyle management
NAICS	North American Industry Classification System
NCSS	National Computer Security Survey
OHS	occupational health services
OMB	Office of Management and Budget
OSH	Occupational Safety and Health
PMPM	per person per month
ROI	return on investment
SIC	Standard Industrial Classification

Chapter 1: Introduction

1.1. Chronic Disease as a Public Health Issue

Over the last several decades, an epidemic of "lifestyle diseases" has been developing in the United States (Pollard, 2008). The Centers for Disease Control and Prevention (CDC) identified four behaviors—inactivity, poor nutrition, tobacco use, and frequent alcohol consumption—as primary causes of chronic disease in the United States, resulting in increasing prevalence of diabetes, heart disease, and chronic pulmonary conditions (Centers for Disease Control and Prevention, 2010). These chronic conditions have become a major burden in the United States, as they lead to decreased quality of life (Healthy People 2020, 2011) and premature death and disability (Centers for Disease Control and Prevention, 2010).

Another concern is the cost of treating chronic disease, estimated to account for over 75 percent of national health expenditures (Centers for Disease Control and Prevention, 2010). Furthermore, although chronic disease was once thought to be a problem of older age groups, the number of working-age adults with a chronic condition has grown by 25 percent in ten years (Hoffman and Schwartz, 2008). This shift toward earlier onset adds to the economic burden of chronic disease because of illness-related loss of productivity resulting from absence from work (absenteeism) and reduced performance while at work (presenteeism). Results from a PricewaterhouseCoopers survey found that indirect costs (e.g., days missed at work) were approximately four times higher for individuals with chronic disease than for those without (PricewaterhouseCoopers, 2010). Moreover, a report released by the Milken Institute estimated that the indirect costs of these illnesses was higher than the direct health care costs to treat chronic disease (DeVol et al., 2007). The cumulative losses associated with chronic disease totaled a startling $1 trillion in 2003, whereas $277 billion was spent on direct health care (DeVol et al., 2007).

1.2. Growing Interest in Wellness Programs among Employers

With the increasing prevalence of chronic diseases in the working-age population, employers are concerned about their effect on the cost of employer-sponsored health coverage and productivity. In a recent survey by benefits consultant Towers Watson and the National Business Group on Health (NBGH), 67 percent of employers identified "employees' poor health habits" as one of their top three challenges to maintaining affordable health coverage (National Business Group on Health, 2010).

To counter the trend of increasing health care costs, employers are adopting health promotion and disease prevention strategies, often referred to as workplace wellness programs (111th Congress, 2010). Disease prevention programs aim either to prevent the onset of diseases (primary prevention) or to diagnose and treat disease at an early stage before complications occur (secondary prevention). Primary prevention addresses health-related behaviors and risk factors—for example, by encouraging a diet with lower fat and caloric content to prevent the onset of diabetes mellitus. Secondary prevention attempts to improve disease control—for example, by promoting medication adherence for patients with asthma to avoid symptom exacerbations that can lead to hospitalization. Health promotion is related to disease prevention in that it aims at fostering better health through behavior change. Workplace wellness takes advantage of employers' access to employees at an age when interventions can still change their long-term health trajectory.

A formal and universally accepted definition for workplace wellness programs has yet to emerge, and the range of benefits offered under this label is broad. In this report, we distinguish three types of activities that can be offered through the employer's health plan or by the employer directly:

- screening activities to identify health risks (e.g., measurement of body weight)
- primary prevention interventions to address manifest health risks, also referred to as lifestyle management (e.g., weight reduction counseling) and secondary prevention to improve control of chronic conditions, also referred to as disease management
- health promotion activities to further healthy lifestyles (e.g., healthy food options in cafeterias)
    - The overall health and wellness strategy of employers can also encompass other benefits related to health and well-being (e.g., occupational health and safety programs), contextual changes (e.g., smoking bans) and the use of incentives to encourage the uptake of workplace wellness benefits. Those incentives can be tied to program participation (referred to as participatory programs) or to changes in health-related standards, such as smoking or body weight (referred to as health-contingent programs (*Federal Register*, 2012).

The breadth of employers' workplace wellness strategies can vary substantially, from offering vouchers to join a gym to implementing multi-component programs that combine screening, interventions, and changes to the overall benefit design. Additionally, workplace wellness programs and wellness incentive programs as part of those might be offered directly by an employer as a benefit for all employees or as part of an employer-sponsored group health plan for participants and beneficiaries.[7]

Early proponents of workplace interventions, such as Johnson & Johnson, developed their own programs. The emergence of a workplace wellness industry in recent years now allows employers to procure ready-made programs and interventions and has contributed to the uptake of those programs, as they demonstrate favorable results. For example, a recent review conducted meta-analyses of studies that looked at the return on investment (ROI) of wellness programs. It found the ROI to be 3:1 for direct medical cost and also 3:1 for absenteeism (Baicker, Cutler and Song, 2010). However, those positive findings have to be viewed cautiously, because they are typically derived from selected employers with strong commitments to wellness and may not generalize to other employers

But the positive reports have led many employers to regard workplace wellness programs as an effective tool to contain health care costs and, thus, as a viable business strategy. More than half (52 percent) of all employers that offered wellness programs in 2012 believed that they were effective in reducing the firm's health care costs, according to a survey by the Kaiser Family Foundation and the Health Research and Educational Trust (KFF/HRET) (KFF/HRET, 2012). In addition to employers, health insurance issuers are increasingly incorporating wellness programs into their coverage products. The same KFF/HRET survey indicates that among employers with fewer than 200 employees that offered wellness programs, 59 percent did so because the programs were part of the insurance coverage provided by their health plan (KFF/HRET, 2012).

1.3. Role of the Patient Protection and Affordable Care Act
The Affordable Care Act has numerous provisions intended to contain health care cost growth and expand health promotion and prevention activities. For example, it establishes a technical assistance role for the CDC to provide tools and resources to assist employers with implementation planning and

---

[7] Distinguishing whether a program is part of a group health plan can be difficult, but the distinction is important when determining what regulatory provisions may apply. This study attempts to parse out this detail when possible; however the data do not always allow for this. When the distinction is possible, it is noted in the findings. As well, such phrases as "employer-offered" or "employer-sponsored" are used generally throughout this report; however, unless noted otherwise, these phrases should not be read to indicate whether a program is or is not part of a group health plan.

conducting evaluations [8] (Section 4303 of the Affordable Care Act). In addition, the Department of Health and Human Services (DHHS) will award $10 million from the Affordable Care Act's Prevention and Public Health Fund to organizations with expertise in working with employers to develop and expand workplace wellness activities, such as tobacco-free policies, flextime for physical activity, and healthier food choices in the workplace. [9]

Section 2705 (j)(3) of the Public Health Service Act, as amended by the Affordable Care Act, also raises the permissible limit on rewards offered through a group health plan for participating in a wellness program that requires meeting health-related standards (health-contingent programs). This provision gives employers greater latitude in rewarding group health plan participants and beneficiaries for healthy lifestyles through wellness programs that meet certain standards. The limit, currently set at 20 percent of the cost of coverage, will increase to 30 percent in 2014, and the Secretaries of Labor, Health and Human Services, and the Treasury may increase the reward to up to 50 percent if they determine that such an increase is appropriate. [10] These rewards may be provided in such forms as premium discounts, waivers of cost-sharing requirements, or improved benefits. These limits apply only to incentives requiring that individuals meet a health-related standard, such as target body weight, and which are administered under an employment-based group health plan, irrespective of whether the incentives take the form of a reward, a penalty, or a combination of both. Incentives that are not tied to a health factor and are offered to all similarly situated individuals do not have to comply with the requirements of Section 2705(j)(3) of the Public Health Service Act, but must still comply with other applicable federal laws, such as the Genetic Information and Nondiscrimination Act (GINA) and the Americans with Disabilities Act (ADA), and state laws. In addition, the Affordable Care Act includes preventive and wellness services and chronic disease management in its list of essential health benefits that certain health plans will need to offer as of 2014 and specifies that certain recommended preventive services must be covered without cost-sharing as of September 23, 2010. [11]

---

[8] For example, the National Healthy Worksite program is has been funded under the Affordable Care Act to support employers in their efforts to promote health at the workplace (www.cdc.gov/nationalhealthyworksite).

[9] This funding was announced by DHHS in June 2011. See U.S. Department of Health and Human Services (2011).

[10] The Departments of Health and Human Services, Labor, and the Treasury issued a Notice for Proposed Rulemaking regarding incentives for nondiscriminatory wellness programs in group health plans on November 26, 2012 (*Federal Register*, 2012). Final rules regarding incentives for nondiscriminatory wellness programs in group health plans are being contemporaneously published with this report (*Federal Register*, 2013).

[11] "Grandfathered" health insurance plans, which were in existence before passage of the Affordable Care Act, are exempt from those requirements.

1.4. Overview and Research Questions

This report addresses Section 2705(m)(1) of the Public Health Service Act, which requires a survey of national worksite health policies and programs to assess employer-based health policies and programs and a report to Congress that includes recommendations for the implementation of effective employer-based health policies and programs. In this context, the overarching goal of this project is to assess the effectiveness and impact of workplace wellness programs and to identify best practices and lessons learned in program implementation to maximize their impact. A particular focus is studying the effect of employee incentives on program participation and results. The research under this project encompasses collection and analysis of data on the types of wellness programs offered by employers in the United States, employee incentives and their effectiveness and the impact on employee behavior, the affordability of coverage, and health outcomes. The project uses four main data sources:

- a review of the scientific and trade literature to identify the prevalence of wellness programs, their key components, their use of incentives, and the effectiveness of wellness programs' return on investment, and best practices
- a national survey of employers from the public and private sectors, including federal and state agencies, to assess the prevalence, type of wellness programs, information on incentives, and perceived program impact
- statistical analyses using medical and pharmacy claims data and wellness program data from a sample of employers to assess the effects of wellness programs on health and cost outcomes and of incentives on program participation and impact.
- case studies of existing wellness programs in a heterogeneous set of employers to enhance understanding of the impact and effectiveness of wellness programs by providing specific examples and experiences of individuals.

Chapter 2 contains a detailed description of data and methods. We then present our analysis using a thematic approach that integrates findings from the four data sources to address the following topics, reflecting the Affordable Care Act requirements (111th Congress, 2010):

- What are the characteristics and prevalence of current workplace wellness programs? (Chapter 3)
  - What percentage of employers offers a workplace wellness program?

- How are programs configured?

- How do program characteristics vary by industry, firm size, region, and other factors?

- What is the evidence related to program impact? (Chapter 4)

    - To what degree are programs used by employees?

    - What is the effectiveness of wellness programs (as defined in subsection [j]) in promoting health and preventing disease (Section 2705)? (111th Congress, 2010)

    - What impact do such wellness programs have on access to care and the affordability of coverage for participants and nonparticipants of such programs (Section 2705)? (111th Congress, 2010)

- What is the role of incentives under wellness programs? (Chapter 5)

    - What are the current practices of using employee incentives?

    - What is the impact of premium-based and cost-sharing incentives on participant behavior and the role of such programs in changing behavior (Section 2705)? (111th Congress, 2010)

    - What is the effectiveness of different types of rewards (Section 2705)? (111th Congress, 2010)

    - Do incentives have any unintended consequences?

- What are key facilitators of successful wellness programs? (Chapter 6)

Each chapter contains a summary of our findings and an interpretation of those findings in light of the existing literature. The final chapter summarizes the implications of the study and points out a future research agenda.

Chapter 2: Methods

2.1. Literature Review

We conducted a review of the scientific and trade literature and analyses of survey findings on the characteristics and prevalence of workplace wellness programs. The scientific literature was used primarily to collect evidence on the impact of these programs on health-related behaviors, health outcomes, and cost savings. Before conducting the search, we consulted with experts in government and academia and with representatives of employers, employer organizations, benefits consultancies, and program vendors. A detailed description of the literature review and a full account of our findings have been published in a separate report and a journal article (Mattke, Schnyer and Van Busum, 2012; Osilla et al., 2012).

2.2. RAND Employer Survey

2.2.1. Sampling Frame

The sampling approach for the employer survey had the goal of generating a nationally representative sample of employers to allow us to obtain valid, credible, and reasonably bounded estimates for policy-relevant questions, such as the prevalence of different types of program elements and the types of incentives used to encourage program use.

To generate nationally representative estimates of wellness program use, we drew a stratified random sample that ensured a balanced representation of different types of employers. We created a sampling frame using Dun & Bradstreet (D&B)[12] data that was used to draw a stratified random sample of employers, including private companies and government agencies. We decided to stratify by size and industry, because those company characteristics tend to determine the type and scope of wellness program offerings according to the literature and expert input. We classified industry by the four main categories of the 2007 NAICS: heavy industry (e.g., agriculture, mining, construction, and

---

[12] The D&B database contains a complete listing of private and public companies or organizations in the United States. It was used previously for the Annual Employer Health Benefits Survey by (KFF/HRET, 2010) As of the end of 2011 when the sample was drawn, the D&B database had records on 72.4 million businesses and government agencies. It provides information on the organizations that allows generation of a stratified sample and pre-populating certain data points on corporate structure. For example, variables are available on whether a company has one or multiple locations, whether it is a branch or the headquarters, whether it is a subsidiary or a parent company, and which company is its branch, subsidiary, or parent company. The database also provides industry classification systems, such as Standard Industrial Classification (SIC) or North American Industry Classification System (NAICS) codes, employment size, and contact information for a variety of key personnel in each company. Furthermore, D&B creates a unique nine-digit identifier, the Data Universal Numbering System (DUNS) number, for each company, which will be retained for a company even if it goes out of business.

manufacturing), trade (e.g., retail trade and warehousing), service (e.g., information, finance and insurance, and educational services), and public administration (e.g., federal and state governments) (NAICS, 2011). Size was categorized by number of employees: ≥ 50 and ≤ 100 workers, > 100 and ≤ 1,000 workers, > 1,000 and ≤ 10,000 workers, > 10,000 and < 50,000 workers, and > 50,000 workers. We excluded employers with fewer than 50 workers, because they are subject to different regulations.[13]

The starting sample included 3,000 unique D&B entries and was designed to maximize the informational yield of the collected data. We used the 2010 KFF/HRET Health Benefits Survey as a benchmark, because this survey is commonly used as the source of nationally representative estimates on benefits, especially health insurance offerings. With a sample of 3,143 firms, the KFF/HRET survey is considerably larger than those conducted by consultancies and employer associations that tend to include fewer than 1,000 companies (KFF/HRET, 2010).

Combining four industry categories with five categories for firm size yields 20 sampling strata, with, on average, 150 firms selected per strata based on our starting sample size of 3,000 firms. Our power calculation for this initial sample showed that the survey would yield an estimate of program offering rate with a margin of error of 5 percentage points, assuming a response rate of 35 percent, which was based on previous RAND experience with the 2006 National Computer Security Survey (NCSS), a web-based survey with a response rate of 27 percent among firms with 100 or more employees (Davis et al., 2008). Thus, we expected that the initial sample of 3,000 firms would generate sufficiently precise estimates for the purpose of the study. The details of statistical power calculation and sample allocation are described in Appendix A.

2.2.2. Survey Methods

We developed a survey questionnaire based on the published literature and prior surveys, such as the wellness program section of the KFF/HRET Employer Health Benefits Survey. We ensured that the instrument is easy to read, easy to navigate, and contains open spaces between items. We developed

---

[13] For example, the Affordable Care Act exempts them from penalties if they do not offer health insurance coverage, and most states consider them part of the small group market. They typically have a different range of health-related benefits, as the small group market has less sophisticated insurance products and lower coverage rates. Use of wellness programs tends to be lower and customization of programs rare. This restriction excludes 98 percent of employers but only 25 percent of the total workforce (Hoovers: A Dun & Bradstreet Company, undated).

the instrument in both paper and web-based formats to meet these criteria. The final instrument includes the following sections: introduction, wellness program overview, health risk assessment, lifestyle or risk factor management, incentives for health results, clinical screening, disease management, program evaluation and costs, other employee benefits, employer background, and a section for employers without a wellness program. The instrument is 19 pages long and the estimated completion time is about 30 minutes.

We performed cognitive testing of the survey questions by conducting nine 90-minute interviews with employer representatives, including one general manager, five human resource managers, and three employee benefits managers. The interviewees came from employers with 140 to 34,000 employees. The purpose of this testing was to test the content of the questions, the ease of navigation, and the appropriateness or "fit" of response categories to response tasks. In each interview, respondents completed the survey questionnaire, and we conducted follow-up or cognitive probes. The survey instrument was revised based on their responses and feedback.

To obtain Office of Management Budget (OMB) clearance, we worked with the task order officers and prepared a 60-day *Federal Register* notice required by the Paperwork Reduction Act of 1995, before the submission of an OMB Clearance Package. We responded to public comments generated by the 60-day *Federal Register* notices as appropriate. These procedures ensured that all comments were addressed and prevented duplication of effort to respond to the same or similar comments from different sources. A package, including the survey instrument, the key informant guide, the focus group protocol, a 30-day *Federal Register* notice, and all survey materials (e.g., letters, emails, and introductory telephone script) was submitted to the OMB.

The data were primarily collected using a web-based survey, but we mailed paper versions on request. We also made a PDF version of the questionnaire available for download on the website and conducted one follow-up mailing of paper copies of the survey to nonrespondents. Using the Dun & Bradstreet database, we identified a company representative who would be likely to respond to the web-based survey (e.g., a benefits manager or human resource representative) and contacted the representative via email. We made telephone calls to the sampled employers without such listings to identify the appropriate person. Once an employer contact was identified, we sent that contact an initial invitation by email. If an email address was not available, a letter was sent with the link and password for completing the web-based survey. A reminder letter or email was sent to nonrespondents three weeks after the initial invitation. Approximately three weeks after the reminder letter or email was sent, if the employer had not completed the web-based survey and had not already been removed from the sample (e.g., refusal), a paper survey was mailed to the contact. Telephone calls were made to employers who had not completed the survey, with a special focus on the strata with high nonresponse rates.

We adopted the following strategies to maximize the response rate. First, we drew the sample close to the actual fielding of the survey to assure that the posted contact information was current. Further, we made the instrument user-friendly and simplified questions. The web-based instrument was estimated to take no more than 30 minutes to complete, including the time it may take respondents to look up and retrieve required information. Moreover, the survey methodology included follow-up with nonrespondents to maximize response rates, such as sending prompting letters, emails, or a paper copy of the questionnaire and conducting telephone follow-ups for employers who had not responded to requests. The overall response rate among all sampled employers was 19 percent, with variation by employer size and industry category (see Table A.4). Comparisons between respondents and nonrespondents show some patterns in survey responses. For example, government agencies and smaller employers were both more likely to respond to the survey. Employers with fewer years in business or those who were a subsidiary of another company were found to be less likely to respond (see Table A.6). These comparisons of survey respondents and nonrespondents do not allow us to determine whether employers with a wellness program were more or less likely to respond to the survey.

We used the KFF/HRET survey (KFF/HRET, 2012) to inform our decisions on the target sample size and data source for the sample, as it is a commonly referenced source of information on employer-sponsored health benefits, but we tailored our survey to our research questions. First, we asked more detailed questions on wellness program components and incentive use than does the KFF survey, which asks about various types of employer-sponsored health benefits. Second, we used a sample frame based on the likelihood of wellness program offering rather than the overall universe of employers used for the KFF/HRET survey, included federal government agencies, and used four industry categories and five employment size categories, whereas the KFF/HRET survey used ten industry categories and six size categories. Third, we excluded employers with 50 or fewer employees, because they are subject to different regulations (see Appendix A for details), whereas the KFF/HRET survey targets employers with at least three employees. Last, the KFF/HRET survey is a telephone survey and our survey is web-based

2.2.3. Data Analysis

As the first step, we identified companies in each stratum that had gone out of business or ceased to exist as independent companies and adjusted the sampling frame (the population size). To account for nonresponse, a final sampling weight was calculated for each of the 20 strata as the product of the initial sampling weight and the reciprocal of the weighted response rate (see Appendix A for details). Although some respondents completed only part of the questionnaire, we considered their responses valid if they answered all the five key questions about program offerings: any wellness program, Health Risk Assessment (HRA), screening, lifestyle management, and disease management. For item nonresponse, we substituted missing values only when the missing information could be derived from a respondent's answers to other questions. For example, if an employer did not answer whether a specific wellness program was offered but answered questions about the wellness program, such as which incentives were used and what the average participation rate was, we indicated that the employer had that specific wellness program. The final response rate of the survey was 19 percent (see Appendix A for details), a typical response rate for a business survey using a nontelephone survey mode (KFF/HRET, 2010). All reported results are based on final sampling weights adjusted for nonresponse and are therefore generalizable at the national level.

2.3. Employer Case Studies

2.3.1. Selection of Employers

Case study candidates were identified from published information, such as companies listed in the Partnership for Prevention "Leading by Example" publications, highlighted in awards programs (e.g., Wellness Councils of America Awards and C. Everett Koop Awards), featured in newspaper articles, and/or referred to us by experts on worksite wellness programs. We attempted to recruit sites that had well-established programs and that differ along the following criteria:

- company size
- type of employer (heavy industry, retail, services, and government)
- program origin ("home-grown" versus offered by a health plan or vendor)
- region of the country.

In total, we identified 34 candidate employers for the case studies based on our selection criteria. We selected primary and backup sites to achieve balanced representation of our selection criteria. Nine organizations were contacted to secure participation from four employers.

Two primary sites agreed to participate and the other two sites were recruited from the backup list. In addition, we used data that we collected during a recent site visit under a separate study (see Table 2.1).

Of note, we were unable to secure participation of any small firm with less than 1,000 employees, even though we had identified and contacted three candidate organizations. Representatives of these firms felt that the burden of study participation would be too high for their employees, company management was reluctant to participate, or no staff was available to help with study coordination.

2.3.2. Data Collection

Each case study was based on data collected through semi-structured interviews with key informants, focus groups with program participants, and direct observation. We developed a semi-structured interview protocol to guide expert interviews. The questions were informed by a literature review and expert consultations. We conducted individual interviews with wellness program coordinators, wellness program staff, human resource representatives, accountants, worker representatives, and senior executives. If appropriate, we also interviewed benefits consultants, health plan staff, and program vendor representatives.

Each case study also included at least one employee focus group to get the end-user perspective on the impact and effectiveness of the wellness program. As with the key informant discussion guides, the focus group protocol was informed by the literature review.

In addition, researchers reviewed relevant, published materials about wellness programs provided by sites themselves. Examples of these materials include brochures describing the wellness program to employees, internal studies documenting the program's effectiveness, peer-reviewed publications about the program, or any literature provided to employees. All data collection and analysis procedures were reviewed and approved by RAND's Institutional Review Board.

Table 2.1. Characterization of Case Study Employers

	Number of Employees	Industry	Region	Contributors to Program Administration
Employer A	3,500	Services	South	Health plan; employer
Employer B	19,000	Government	South	Health plan; employer
Employer C	4,800	Services	Northeast	Health plan; vendor; employer
Employer D	9,000	Manufacturing	Midwest	Health plan; vendor; employer
Employer E	62,000	Government	South and Midwest	Employer; vendor

2.3.3. Analysis

The qualitative data collected from each case study were analyzed thematically by the team that conducted the respective site visit. After all interviews and focus groups were transcribed, researchers reviewed the transcripts to ensure accuracy. Interview and focus group guides were used to facilitate data coding, ensure coding consistency across case studies, and produce comparable individual case study reports. Such an approach to qualitative data analysis helped us ensure that similar data were abstracted for each case study, which is important for synthesizing information across all five case studies and illustrating the main study findings.

2.4. Analysis of Secondary Data from Wellness Programs

2.4.1. Data Source

The data source for this portion of the project is the Data Aggregation Project, a collaboration between the RAND Corporation, the Care Continuum Alliance (CCA), which is the trade organization of the health and wellness management industry, and a database vendor. This project compiles in an anonymized fashion a convenience sample of data from health and wellness management companies and the employers whom they serve for research purposes. The following types of data are collected in standardized formats:

- health plan enrollment data, including employee age, gender, insurance type, and state of residence
- medical and prescription claims

- HRA data (i.e., self-reported health risks and health-related behaviors, such as smoking and exercise)
- biometric screening data (e.g., cholesterol level, body mass index)
- data on employee participation in health and wellness programs
- employer characteristics, such as incentives for program uptake, industry, employment size, average employee compensation, leadership support for wellness programs, and geographic location.

To date, the database contains data from seven large employers with an employment size ranging from about 8,000 to 145,000, covering years 2005 to 2010. The database currently includes about 567,506 unique employees and about 1.8 million employee years. Because of limited data, we had to exclude two employers from the analysis, resulting in a final sample of 362,136 unique employees and 1.2 million employee years. The employers are not identified in the database and do not overlap with the employers in our case studies.

2.4.2. Outcomes of Interest

Medical cost was measured using allowed charges on claims data, including inpatient, outpatient, and prescription claims. Following the literature in wellness program research, we used per-member per-month (PMPM) cost as the outcome. All cost measures were adjusted for inflation. Measures of health care use include emergency department visits per 1,000 employee years and inpatient admissions per 1,000 employee years.

Health behavior outcomes include smoking status and exercise based on data availability. Both outcomes are self-reported as part of the HRA. Smoking status is a dichotomous outcome, measured as either a yes or no response to a question asking about current cigarette smoking. Exercise was measured as the number of days per week of at least 20 minutes of exercise. The Centers for Disease Control and Prevention recommend a minimum of 150 minutes of exercise for adults per week for important health benefits (Centers for Disease Control and Prevention, 2011). This roughly corresponds to at least 20 minutes of exercise daily using the definition of exercise in the HRA data in our analyses.

Health status measures include Body Mass Index (BMI) and total cholesterol, which are from HRA data and clinical screenings. We were not able to examine other health status measures because of limited health status information in HRA. BMI is a ratio of body weight (in kilograms) over squared height (in meters). When BMI is between 25 and 30, a person is considered overweight; a BMI of 30 or greater indicates obesity. Total cholesterol is measured in mg/dL; a total cholesterol level of 200 to 239 is considered borderline high cholesterol, and a cholesterol level of 240 or greater reflects high cholesterol.

2.4.3. Exposures of Interest

<u>Program Participation</u>

Program participation was defined as actual engagement with the program. Specifically, an employee was considered to be a participant only when she or he had at least one phone or mail contact with the wellness program.

<u>Incentives</u>

Incentives were measured as the overall difference in the monetary benefit that a full-time employee can experience per year for engaging in wellness programs, through participation in screenings or interventions, and through health goal attainment. For the calculation of incentive value, we did not distinguish whether incentives were framed as rewards or as penalties or in which form the incentive was paid (e.g., cash, premium differentials). Employers were asked to provide the monetary value of noncash incentives (e.g., gym membership) when applicable.

Table 2.2 shows the incentives (by type) offered by the five employers in our incentives analytic sample for the years used in our analyses. In this sample, HRA incentives are offered to employees for completing an HRA. Incentives for lifestyle management (LM) typically require completing at least one coaching session. Most often, LM incentives are available only to employees who are determined to be "eligible" for a given LM component (i.e., their HRA results indicated the presence of relevant health risks).

2.4.4. Analytic Methods

To address the two key research questions for the secondary data analysis, we compared program participants and nonparticipants using the following strategies:

Table 2.2: Incentives Offered by Employers in the CCA Analytic sample, by Year

Employer	Incentive Type		2006	2007	2008	2009	2010
				Incentive Amount ($)			
1	HRA		0	0	75	75	75
	LM		0	0	125	125	75
		Total	0	0	200	200	150
2	HRA		0	0	0	50	0
	LM		0	0	0	50	0
		Total	0	0	0	100	0
3	HRA		0	0	0	100	100
	LM		0	0	0	0	100
		Total	0	0	0	100	200
4	HRA		0	50	50	50	–
	LM		0	0	0	0	–
		Total	0	50	50	50	–
5	HRA		0	100	100	100	100
	LM		0	100	100	100	100
		Total	0	200	200	200	200

SOURCE: RAND analysis of health plan claims, screening, and wellness program data in the CCA database.
NOTE: "–" denotes that no incentives data are available.

(1) Is program participation associated with changes in outcomes as defined above? To answer this question, we identified employees who were flagged as eligible for wellness program participation based on HRA or screening results and who chose to participate as the intervention group and eligible employees who did not participate as the comparison group. We looked at the differential changes in outcomes between those two groups over time to identify the program effect—the so-called difference-in-differences approach.

(2) Are incentives for program uptake associated with employee engagement and outcomes? To answer this question, we exploited the variation in incentives offered across employers and within employers over time. We examined how the variation in incentives was associated with HRA completion, lifestyle management program participation, health behaviors, and health outcomes.

Thus, the key independent variables, or predictors of interest, were indicators of lifestyle program participation and employee incentives.

Descriptive Analyses

Descriptive analyses were conducted to summarize the characteristics of employers, employees, and wellness programs in the sample. These analyses included means and frequency tabulations. In addition, we describe program participation, duration of participation, trends in medical costs, use of care, health behaviors, and health outcomes among participants and nonparticipants over time. Bivariate relationships between outcomes and key independent variables were also examined. We used appropriate statistical tests, such as t-tests and chi-squared tests, for the bivariate relationships between variables.

Multivariate Analyses

Since nonparticipants may be different from participants in observed and unobserved ways, simply using nonparticipants as the comparison group may yield biased estimates. To account for differences as much as possible in this observational study, we first identified a valid comparison group using propensity score matching and then performed longitudinal regression analysis using the matched pairs. This way, comparison members would be similar to program participants in observed characteristics at baseline. In addition, longitudinal regression analysis was used to account for the unobserved employee characteristics using employee-level fixed effects. The longitudinal analysis generated impact estimates for multiple-year program participation, varying from one year to five years. Despite our analytic approaches to control for both observed and unobserved employee characteristics, there might be some residual bias that could potentially affect our parameter estimates, such as differential changes in employees' motivation to improve their health. As a result, our findings should be interpreted with caution. See additional details in Appendix B.

Simulation Analyses to Demonstrate Cumulative Program Impact

Since workplace wellness programs are multiyear interventions that are expected to achieve benefits over time, we sought to devise an intuitive way to estimate and present cumulative program impact based on the regression results. Basically, we took a hypothetical cohort of employees who are representative of the estimation sample. We used this cohort to simulate outcomes as if they participated in the program (intervention cohort); similarly, we used the same cohort to simulate outcomes as if they did not participate (comparison cohort). We then applied estimated program effects as well as secular trends in outcomes derived from regressions to demonstrate cumulative program impacts. (See additional details in Appendix B.)

Chapter 3: Employer-Based Wellness Program Characteristics and Prevalence

Chapter 3 examines current program uptake among employers and the composition of currently deployed workplace wellness programs. Using findings from the RAND Employer Survey and our case studies, we describe the availability of worksite wellness benefits, such as *wellness screening activities* like HRAs or onsite clinical screenings and *interventions* designed to promote health-related behaviors (lifestyle management) and manage manifest disease (disease management).

3.1. Availability of Employer-Based Wellness Programs

The RAND Employer Survey data suggest that nationally, about half (51 percent) of all employers with 50 or more employees offer a wellness program,[14] ranging between 44 percent of heavy industry employers and 66 percent of government employers, although this difference is not statistically significant (Figure 3.1).

Figure 3.1: Percentage of Employers Offering a Wellness Program, by Industry

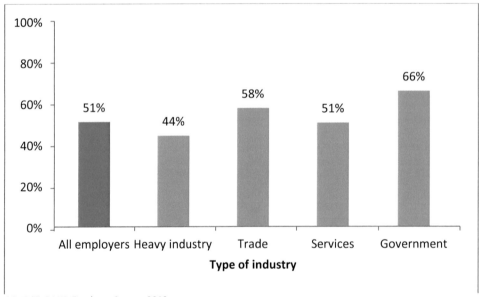

SOURCE: RAND Employer Survey, 2012.
NOTES: The graph represents information from employers with at least 50 employees. There is no significant difference in the distribution of wellness programs (p > 0.05).

---

[14] Among employers offering health insurance benefits to active full-time employees, 57 percent provide a wellness program.

Larger employers are more likely to have wellness programs (p < 0.01). As shown in Figure 3.2, the percentage of large employers (> 1,000 employees) having a wellness program is more than twice that of the smallest employers in our sample (50 to 100 employees).

Although only about half of all employers offer wellness programs, more than three-quarters (79 percent) of employees working for firms and organizations with 50 or more employees have access to a wellness program, because large employers, who account for a greater share of the workforce, are more likely to have such programs (Figure 3.3).[15]

Employers' likelihood of offering wellness programs ranges from 66 percent in the Northeast to 42 percent in the West, although this difference was not significant (Figure 3.4).

Figure 3.2: Percentage of Employers Offering a Wellness Program, by Employer Size

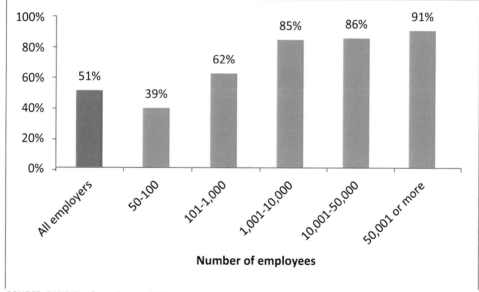

SOURCE: RAND Employer Survey, 2012.
NOTES: The graph represents information from employers with at least 50 employees. There is a significant difference in the distribution of wellness programs (p < 0.01).

---

[15] Data source: 10,000 sample of the Dun & Bradstreet business database of firms in the United States with at least 50 employees. For each of the 20 strata, we calculated the number of employees with access to a wellness program by multiplying the prevalence of wellness programs (from the survey results) * mean number of employers * number of firms; the numerator is equal to the summation of the 20 strata totals. We calculated the total number of employees for each strata by multiplying the mean number of employers * number of firms; the denominator is equal to the summation of the 20 strata totals.

Figure 3.3: Estimated Percentage of Employees at Firms and Organizations with 50 or More Employees with Access to a Wellness Program

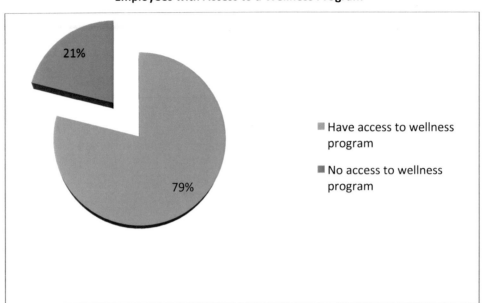

Figure 3.4: Percentage of Employers Offering a Wellness Program, by Geographic Region

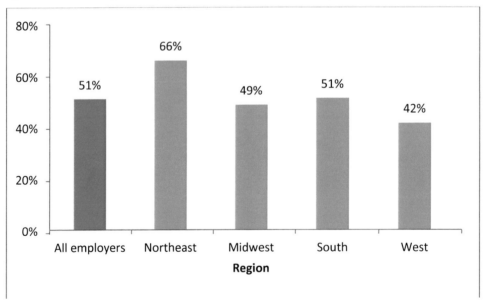

SOURCE: RAND Employer Survey, 2012.
NOTES: The graph represents information from employers with at least 50 employees. There was no significant difference in the distribution of wellness programs (p > 0.05).

About half of employers do not offer a wellness program, of which almost all (91 percent) had not offered a program in the past five years. Employers indicated absence of cost-effectiveness, lack of resources, and low interest from both management and employees as reasons for not offering a program. Three-quarters of employers who had recently discontinued their program cited the lack of financial resources as an important reason for cancellation. Overall, about a quarter of employers (27 percent) without a wellness program were considering introducing one in the near future.

3.2. Wellness Program Components[16]

A formal and universally accepted definition for workplace wellness programs has yet to emerge, and the range of benefits offered under this label is broad. In this report, we distinguish three types of activities:

- *screening activities* to identify health risks (e.g., measurement of body weight)
- *preventive interventions* to address manifest health risks (e.g., weight-reduction counseling)
- *health promotion activities* to further healthy lifestyles (e.g., healthy food options in cafeterias).

In addition, employers offer other benefits related to health and well-being (e.g., occupational health and safety programs).

3.2.1. Screening Activities

Employer-based wellness programs often include screening activities to identify health risks, most commonly the HRA and biometric screening. An HRA (or health risk questionnaire) is a self-administered questionnaire used to collect information about common modifiable risk factors about behaviors and characteristics, such as nutrition, physical activity, smoking, cholesterol levels, weight, and blood pressure. Biometric, or clinical, screening collects data on height, weight, resting heart rate, blood pressure, blood glucose levels (for diabetes), and blood lipid levels (e.g., cholesterol). Some employers offer additional tests based on clinical guidelines, such as the cancer screening based on recommendations of the U.S. Preventive Services Task Force. These screenings can be conducted at the workplace, in occupational health or primary care clinics, or in partnership with health plans through the employees' regular physicians. The RAND Employer Survey results suggest that almost two-thirds (65 percent) of employers with a wellness program use HRAs, and almost half (49 percent) of them conduct biometric screenings.

---

[16] To minimize the burden on survey respondents, we did not ask them to point out which components of their wellness program were administered by the employer, by its health plans, or by third-party vendors.

3.2.2. Preventive Interventions

Wellness programs offer primary prevention interventions to reduce health risks, referred to as lifestyle management, and secondary prevention interventions to prevent disease exacerbation, referred to as disease management. More than three-quarters (77 percent) of employers with a wellness program offer lifestyle management and over half (56 percent) offer disease management (Figure 3.5). Lifestyle or risk factor management programs are interventions designed to help workers make positive changes to their health-related behaviors. These interventions may be offered to all employees, such as through educational campaigns, or individually administered, such as by counseling. They promote health-related behaviors, such as improved nutrition, more exercise, and smoking cessation. For instance, employees may be encouraged to increase physical activity with so-called step-counting programs that motivate employees to build more walking into their daily routines. Similarly, employers may educate employees about the health risks of obesity and smoking and provide coaching interventions to address those risks.

Whereas lifestyle management programs aim to prevent chronic illness, disease management programs target employees living with chronic diseases, such as heart disease, diabetes, and asthma. Such disease management programs can be offered through an employer's health plan or by a separate program vendor and can be integrated with other program components. These programs are individually targeted and provide ongoing support for issues related to chronic illness, such as medication adherence. They are likely to require long-term engagement with the employee and coordination with the employee's regular physician. For these reasons, disease management programs are often operated separately from the short-term behavioral interventions under lifestyle management.

3.2.3. Health Promotion Activities

A variety of health promotion activities can be offered as part of an employer's wellness program. As outlined above, those benefits are meant to encourage healthy lifestyles and are usually available to all employees, irrespective of whether they have health risks or manifest disease.

- **on-site vaccination services,** such as for influenza
- **fitness benefits,** such as free or subsidized gym memberships and on-site gyms
- **healthy food options,** for example in cafeterias and vending machines

23

- **nurse advice lines,** which provide employees with access to nurses by telephone to receive confidential health information and advice; services are often available 24 hours a day.

The RAND Employer Survey results show that such health promotion activities have become quite common. Half of all employers, including those stating that they do not have a formal wellness program, offer on-site vaccinations, and over 40 percent have a fitness benefit. Other offerings are less common, but the breadth of potential benefits illustrates the variety of approaches that employers take to improve the health and well-being of their workforce. If the sample is restricted to employers with wellness programs, the patterns of additional wellness-related benefits offerings are similar, but rates of provision are higher (Figure 3.5). For example, three-quarters of employers with wellness programs also offer on-site vaccinations. As part of their health promotion activities, employers sometimes make changes to the physical environment of the workplace as part of their wellness strategy, such as making stairs accessible and installing bike racks or walking paths. For example, 13 percent of all employers and

Figure 3.5: Rates of Prevention and Health Promotion Activities Offered by Employers with Wellness Programs

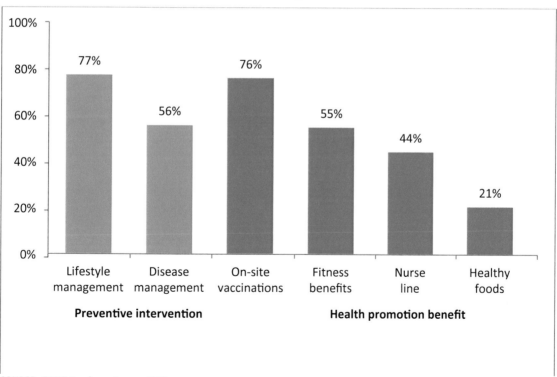

SOURCE: RAND Employer Survey, 2012.
NOTE: This graph represents information from the subset of employers with at least 50 employees that offer a wellness program (51 percent).
^aIncludes onsite facilities or discounts, fitness breaks, other exercise opportunities.

22 percent of employers with a wellness program stated that they provided informal exercise opportunities, such as walking trails and inviting staircases.

3.2.4. Other Benefits Related to Health and Well-Being

In addition to the wellness program components, a variety of other benefits related to health and well-being can be offered as part of an employer's overall wellness strategy:

- **employee assistance programs (EAP):** An EAP provides access to counseling and assistance for personal issues that can have a negative impact on the employee's ability to be focused and productive at work. EAP vendors can offer brief interventions or referrals to community resources—for example, for stress relief, mental health problems, or substance abuse. They also address "work-life balance" issues, such as time management, and offer resources for nonwork responsibilities, such as child or elder care.

- **occupational health services (OHS)**: OHS programs aim to prevent injury in the workplace and may provide onsite clinics for certain health conditions, such as back pain. Although directly related to employee health, they are often managed from a safety and compliance perspective and are subject to a different regulatory framework.

- **on-site clinics:** Some employers now maintain on-site health clinics so that workers can seek certain types of care without leaving the workplace. These clinics vary widely in terms of staffing and scope. They may be staffed by nurses, nurse practitioners and physician assistants, and sometimes by physicians. They typical typically focus on occupational health, including diagnosis, noncomplex treatment, and referral for work-related injury and illness. Employers are increasingly offering a wider array of primary care services at these clinics, including preventive screenings, disease management, and urgent care.[11]

- **absenteeism management:** Some companies have implemented programs to more actively manage employees' return to work from short-term disability leave. These programs are intended to help employees minimize time spent away from work following injuries or illnesses. Employers reach out to workers while they are recovering and help to make arrangements that allow workers to return to the workplace, sometimes with modified or restricted duty. By actively managing short-term disability, employers believe that they can reduce costs associated with lost productivity and keep employees from becoming disengaged during their time away from work.

The RAND Employer Survey results show that such benefits have become quite common (Figure 3.6). Over 40 percent of employers, irrespective of whether they stated having a wellness program or not, reported to have an EAP and 24 percent report having an occupational health service. About 5 percent of employers with 50 or more employees nationally maintain an on-site clinic.

3.3. Wellness Program Operation

Most employers (72 percent) characterize their wellness programs as a combination of screening activities and interventions. Screening activities identify health risks at an individual level, to heighten employees' awareness and direct them to appropriate resources. On the population level, wellness screenings are used to understand and track the overall burden of health risks for planning, program evaluation, and risk management purposes.

As Figure 3.7 shows, the majority of employers with wellness programs support both screening and intervention activities. However, some employers offer intervention-only programs, i.e., direct access to interventions without prior screening for health risks.

Figure 3.6: Rates of Wellness-Related Benefits Offered by Employers

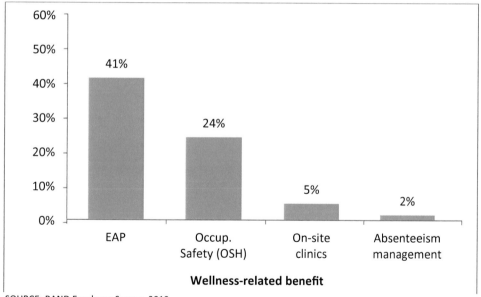

SOURCE: RAND Employer Survey, 2012.
NOTES: The graph represents information from employers with at least 50 employees, regardless of whether they offer a wellness program.

Figure 3.7: Percentage Distribution of Wellness Activities Among Employers with Wellness Programs

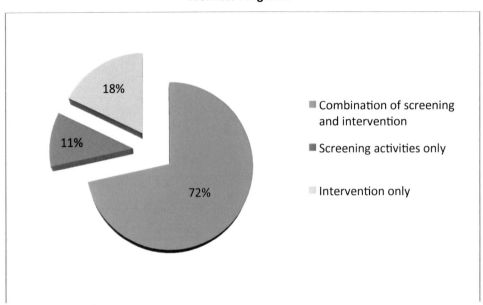

SOURCE: RAND Employer Survey, 2012.
NOTES: This graph represents information from the subset of employers with at least 50 employees that offer a wellness program (51 percent). Percentages do not sum to 100 percent because of rounding.

This result is consistent with the findings from our five case study employers, all of which have a combination of wellness screenings and intervention components, albeit with different degrees of sophistication. Three of the five employers report that they use results from screenings to match employees directly to services that address their health risks. For example, Employer C collects data through biometric screenings, online health risk questionnaires, and analysis of medical claims data. Screenings test for cholesterol levels, blood pressure, blood glucose, and body mass index. Based on the results, an employee may receive a call from a health coach or be linked to ongoing coaching assistance. At some office locations, clinical screenings take place at the workplace, and employees can meet with counselors to develop a customized plan based on their results. Online HRAs, administered by Employer C's health plans, identify individuals who may benefit from behavioral modification or disease management programs and then links them to programs. This employer also receives analyses based on medical and pharmacy claims data from its health plan that point out opportunities to tailor the program to employee needs.

Similarly, Employer E uses an online HRA as a gateway into its wellness programs. Employees are required to register and complete the HRA to be able to access a wellness program. Then they are directed to online content and support resources, based on HRA results. Last, Employer B conducted a pilot program at one of its sites that offered health screening and wellness education during an annual wellness fair. The event, which was held in conjunction with Employee Appreciation Day to make the event more enjoyable and to increase the number of employees who received these screenings, provided employees with an opportunity to discuss their individual results with a medical professional.

3.3.1. Wellness Screening Activities

HRAs are the most common screening method under wellness programs. They are used by over 80 percent of employers with 50 or more employees that conduct any screening (Figure 3.8). A total of 38 percent use only HRAs and 43 percent combine HRAs with clinical screening. In contrast, less than a fifth of all employers collect data only through clinical screening.

Although HRA content has become fairly standardized and includes similar questions (e.g., smoking, exercise, nutrition, weight, stress), our results indicate that clinical screening programs exhibit more variability (Figure 3.9). Blood pressure, glucose, lipids, and BMI are collected by most of these programs to detect metabolic and cardiovascular risks. However, other than these, a wide range of tests are being conducted, such as stress assessment and cancer screening.

Figure 3.8: Percentage Distribution of Screenings Among Employers That Offer Any Screening Activity

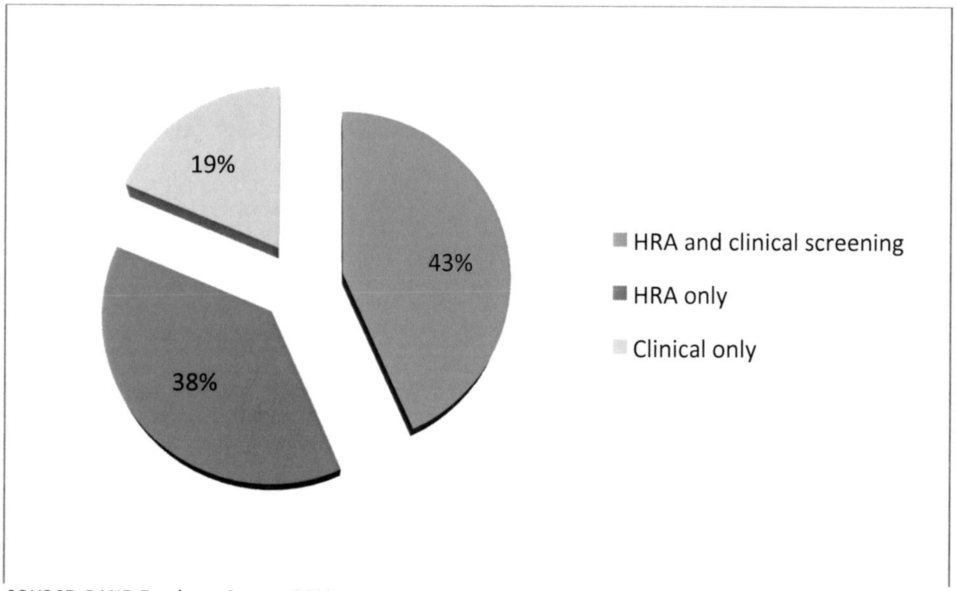

SOURCE: RAND Employer Survey, 2012.
NOTES: The graph represents information from employers with at least 50 employees that offer any screening activity as a component of a wellness program. 51 percent of employers offer a wellness program, and 80 percent have any screening activity.

Figure 3.9: Percentage Distribution of Types of Clinical Screening Tests Offered by Employers That Have Clinical Screenings in Their Wellness Programs

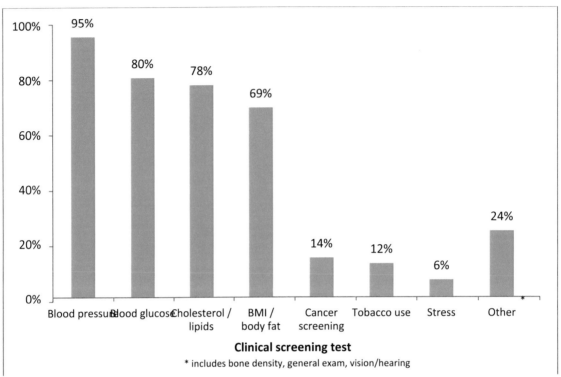

SOURCE: RAND Employer Survey, 2012.
NOTES: The graph represents information from employers with at least 50 employees that offer any clinical screening as a component of a wellness program. 51 percent of employers offer a wellness program, and 49 percent of those include clinical screenings.
[a]Includes bone density, general exam, and vision/hearing tests.

In addition, we learned in our case studies that health plans commonly analyze medical and pharmacy claims data to identify and target employees with manifest chronic conditions for disease management interventions and to spot opportunities to optimize wellness interventions. For example, Employer D's health plan had detected low uptake rates for some screening tests, such as mammograms and colonoscopies, prompting the employer to launch a screening awareness campaign.

3.3.2. Lifestyle Management Programs

As the RAND Employer Survey shows, lifestyle management programs target a broad range of risk factors (Figure 3.10). Given the importance of obesity as driver of chronic disease risk and health care cost, interventions on nutrition, weight, and fitness are offered by about three-quarters of employers. Similarly, although smoking is less common than obesity among employees overall, its substantial impact on health and health care cost explains why 77 percent of employers offer smoking cessation programs. Also common are programs to address substance abuse and manage stress.

Figure 3.10: Percentage Distribution of Types of Lifestyle Management Programs Offered by Employers Providing Any Lifestyle Management Component in Their Wellness Program

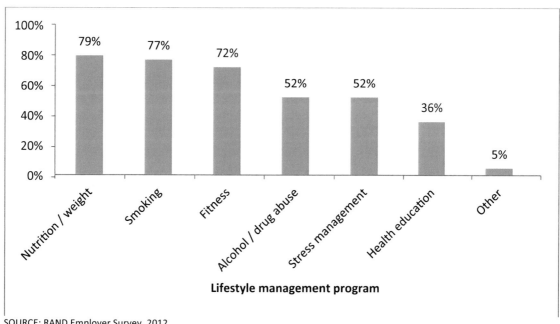

SOURCE: RAND Employer Survey, 2012.
NOTES: The graph represents information from employers with at least 50 employees that offer any lifestyle management intervention as a component of a wellness program. 51 percent of employers offer a wellness program, and 77 percent of those have a lifestyle management intervention.

From our case studies, we learned that programs targeting *nutrition and weight loss* include onsite Weight Watchers group meetings; weight loss competitions (see The Biggest Loser text box); weight loss management programs that offer educational information on nutrition and healthy eating, as well as personalized phone support from health coaches who help participants monitor their eating patterns and health improvements; delivery of nutritious and fresh meals that meet the guidelines of the American Diabetes Association that employees can consume either at work or at home; availability of healthier food options in cafeterias, vending machines, and meetings and parties organized at work; and organization of 30-day fruit and vegetable challenges that encourage employees to eat more fruits and vegetables.

The Biggest Loser: Employer D offers this eight-week weight loss competition inspired by the eponymous television show. Participants weigh in bi-weekly and have their progress monitored throughout the duration of the program. Employees are provided with healthy recipes and links to gym membership discounts through their health plan, and receive tips on how to stay healthy and fit. Competition winners receive awards, such as a paid time off day, a healthy lunch, or sweatshirts, as well as an acknowledgment letter from the company's president.

All of the five case study employers offered *smoking cessation activities,* including counseling, often designed based on the guidelines of the American Cancer Society; educational lectures about the impact of smoking on health; banning smoking in the workplace; and/or distributing free or subsidized smoking cessation products, such as nicotine gum, lozenges, patches, and certain prescription pills.

Exercise programs include both individual and group activities, such as promotion of individualized walking, organized group walking during the lunch hour (see Walk N-Talk text box), walking/running challenges, exercise classes and team sports, and a marathon training program and sponsorship.

> *Walk N-Talk: This monthly event is designed to encourage employees to participate in group walking during the lunch hour and incorporate more physical activity into their daily schedules. Once a month, program participants walk around the site during their lunch break. According to one of the participants, the program also provides "information about distances and places to walk around and things that you can do, how much benefit you can get from a short amount, and . . . [it helps] you track your calorie burn and what you've done."*
> *(Employer A)*

Other lifestyle management offerings include yoga, guided meditation, and massage services that emphasize stress reduction and relaxation. Although they are not commonly offered by employers and are not typically evidence-based, these programs are quite popular among participants. As one interviewee put it, guided meditation helped her "return to the workplace and be more productive, because you are not allowing thoughts and concerns to interfere with the productivity of your work." Employer C began offering confidential webinars for such health topics as depression or stress, "to provide a sense of privacy to individuals."

Wellness programs also encompass *environmental and structural changes* to encourage healthy lifestyles, such as installing sidewalks at the worksite to allow employees to walk a 15-minute loop, conversion of an unused storage space into bike rooms and showers, elimination of smoking break rooms, and calorie labeling in the cafeteria and vending machines (see the following box).

Calorie Labeling in Cafeterias

NOTE: The onsite cafeteria at Employer C clearly labels calories on certain food products and places "call out stickers" on healthy food options.

Interventions can be very specific to the needs of a particular workforce. Employer C recently began offering webinars on stress and depression and an online stress management program to allow reaching its sales force who are rarely in a physical office location. Employer B has also tried to meet the needs of telecommuters but so far has been unsuccessful. One interviewee described her attempts to involve these telecommuters: "My strategy was to have somebody on the [wellness] team who was remote so that maybe they would have some insight into what we could do that would motivate them. But that's very hard, because they are also remote for team meetings and so they feel like they're not really part of the team." This site tried to motivate employees in any location and with any physical ability to participate by challenging them to walk somewhere in the area they live, take a picture, upload the picture, and then others could guess where the picture was taken. "We have come up with challenges where we thought anyone could participate, but had zero participation in it."

3.3.3. Disease Management

A wide variety of conditions is addressed through employer-sponsored disease management programs (Figure 3.11). Diabetes is the most commonly targeted condition (85 percent), but about half of employers also address asthma, COPD, cardiac disorders, depression, and cancer. Over 20 percent of

Figure 3.11: Conditions Targeted by Employers with Any Disease Management Component in Their Wellness Program

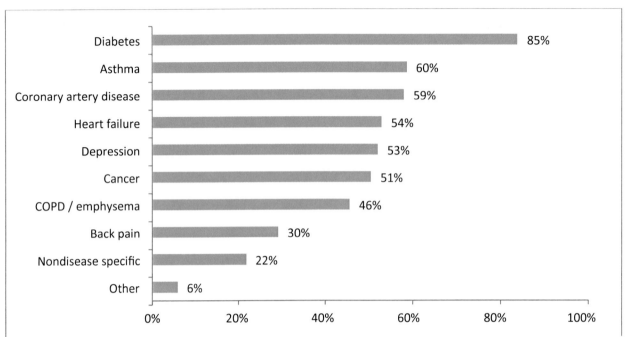

SOURCE: RAND Employer Survey, 2012.
NOTES: The graph represents information from employers with at least 50 employees that offer any disease management intervention as a component of a wellness program. 51 percent of employers offer a wellness program, and 56 percent of those have a disease management intervention.

employers have so-called "holistic programs" that treat patients with chronic conditions in a patient-centric rather than disease-focused manner. "Heavy industry" companies have the highest uptake of disease management programs (70 percent compared to 50–55 percent for the other industries), although this difference is not statistically significant (data not shown).

Results from our case studies suggest that worksite wellness program offerings that help employees manage chronic diseases include individualized health coaching, health lectures and webinars, and wellness fairs that provide both screenings and education for managing such conditions as diabetes or asthma. In our case studies, screenings and health coaching are often provided by health plans, whereas education and lectures are often provided by the employers or vendors. For example, Employer A offers disease management programs through its health plan that provides evidence-based guidelines for screening and treatment, general and targeted outreach, and reminders as well as self-management tools for individuals with chronic conditions. Similarly, case management services and one-on-one nurse coaching to manage a chronic illness or medical event were offered through health plans at three employer sites (B, C, and D). Employees who qualify for disease management programs are identified through an HRA and clinical screenings and then are linked to appropriate services. All five case study employers have provided education and lectures. Employer B has a range of education initiatives including posters, seminars, and bulletin boards. For example, one poster presented an explanation of blood pressure, how you measure it, what the numbers mean, what individuals should watch for, and what one does to follow up if concerned. Employer E offers onsite educational seminars regarding such common diseases as diabetes and asthma. Employers C and D offered onsite seminars for chronic conditions but have since stopped because of low attendance.

The variety of wellness programs offered increases with employer size (p < 0.01). The largest employers (with more than 50,000 employees) consistently offered more types of lifestyle management programs, disease management programs, clinical screenings, and other wellness benefits, such as onsite gym facilities and vaccinations. On average, an employee at the largest companies can choose from over 20 wellness-related offerings, compared to only nine for an employee at the smallest company surveyed (50 to 100 employees) (Figure 3.12).

Figure 3.12: Average Number of Benefits Offered Among Employers with Wellness Programs, by Employer Size

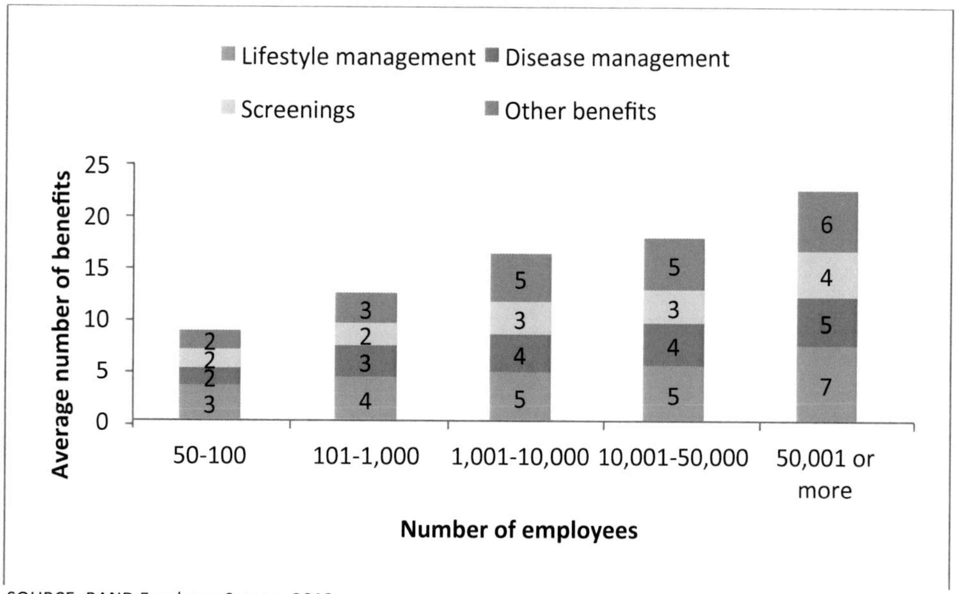

SOURCE: RAND Employer Survey, 2012.
NOTES: The graph represents information from employers with at least 50 employees that offer any wellness program. 51 percent of employers offer a wellness program. There was a significant difference in the number of benefits offered (p < 0.01).

3.4. Discussion of Program Characteristics and Prevalence

The RAND Employer Survey shows that approximately half of U.S. employers with 50 or more employees offer wellness programs (51 percent), across most geographic regions and industries. Larger employers are more likely to have a wellness program and to have more complex programs. These findings are similar to the results from the 2012 KFF/HRET survey, which found that 38 percent of all surveyed employers offered at least one wellness program. [17] It is important to note that the 2012 KFF/HRET survey included employers with three or more employees. Among larger employers (defined in the KFF/HRET survey as those with 200 or more employees), program prevalence was 57 percent (KFF/HRET, 2012), [18] which is consistent with our results. The National Study of Employers, a representative survey by the Families and Work Institute, reported that wellness program offering increased from 51 percent in 1998 to 63 percent in 2012 (Galinsky and Matos, 2012).

Other, nonrepresentative employer surveys indicate that companies continue to be committed to maintaining or expanding their investments in wellness programming despite the economic downturn. PwC Consulting found that 67 percent of employers intended to expand or improve wellness programs in the United States (PricewaterhouseCoopers, 2010), whereas Hewitt Associates reports, based on its 2010 *The Road Ahead* survey, that 42 percent of employers expected to increase their wellness program offerings in spite of the economic downturn (Hewitt Associates, 2010). Similarly, the Integrated Benefits Institute (IBI), a membership organization representing large employers, reports from its 2009 survey that 68 percent of employers planned to expand financial resources devoted to health and productivity management programs (Integrated Benefits Institute, 2010).

Our findings suggest that the most common component of wellness programs is screening activities (HRAs or biometric screening) focused on identifying health risks. Our survey shows that among all employers with 50 or more employees, 33 percent offer an HRA and 25 percent offer clinical screenings. These estimates are similar to those from the 2012 KFF/HRET survey, which suggests that among employers with 200 or more employees, 22 percent offer an HRA and 28 percent offer clinical

---

[17] The 2012 KFF/HRET survey includes public and private firms with three or more employees. Sixty-one percent of employers offered health benefits, and among them, 63 percent offered at least one of the following wellness benefits: weight loss programs, biometric screening, smoking cessation programs, lifestyle or behavioral coaching, gym membership, discounts or on-site exercise facilities, classes in nutrition or healthy living, web-based resources for healthy living, or a wellness newsletter.

[18] The KFF/HRET estimates of program uptake are slightly higher than ours because they include only employers that offer health insurance coverage and those with 200 or more employers, whereas we cover smaller employers ($\geq$ 50 employees), which are less likely to offer wellness programs.

screenings(KFF/HRET, 2012). HRAs tend to be the cornerstone of data collection and are used by about two-thirds of employers with 50 or more employees nationally. Their obvious attraction is that they create a very limited burden on employees, are inexpensive, and can generate data both for matching employees to interventions and for program planning and evaluation.

Our estimates of the prevalence of preventive interventions are very similar to those from the 2012 KFF/HRET survey. Our survey suggests that 39, 31, and 30 percent of employers with 50 or more employees offer a lifestyle management program, a weight control or nutrition program, and a smoking cessation program, respectively, whereas, according to the 2012 KFF/HRET survey, 32, 37, and 40 percent of employers with 200 or more employees have these programs, respectively (KFF/HRET, 2012). Note that the definitions of these programs may differ slightly in the two surveys.

Preventive interventions under worksite wellness programs focus on metabolic and cardiovascular risk factors to prevent diabetes and heart disease and on smoking cessation. This emphasis is mirrored in the conditions that are targeted under disease management programs for employees with such manifest chronic conditions as diabetes, heart disease, and chronic pulmonary conditions. Thus, priority-setting for wellness programs clearly follows disease prevalence trends. In addition, employers customize program offerings to address health risks and conditions that are common in their particular workforce. A variety of other benefits related to health and well-being, such as on-site vaccinations, workplace structural changes, and healthier food options in cafeterias, round out the overall wellness strategy.

To summarize, a clear picture is emerging regarding how employers have incorporated wellness into the workplace in 2012. Wellness *programs* that combine collection of data on health risks with interventions, wellness-related *benefits* such as gym discounts, and *structural changes* to promote healthy behaviors such as accessible staircases, form the overall wellness strategy.

Chapter 4: Program Impact

In Chapter 4, we review the uptake rates of various workplace wellness program components among eligible employees. We then assess evidence of the impacts of workplace wellness programs on health-related behaviors, such as smoking and exercise, and outcomes, such as body weight and blood pressure, as well as the effects on medical costs and health care use. Evidence is drawn from the RAND Employer Survey and CCA database and is supplemented with information from the case studies.

4.1. Program Participation

4.1.1. Wellness Screening

Results from the RAND Employer Survey suggest that about half of employees complete HRAs (46 percent) or participate in clinical screenings (46 percent), if offered, but participation rates for individual employers vary greatly, ranging from 0 to 100 percent. For example, nearly one-third of employers have HRA completion rates of 20 percent or less (Figure 4.1), whereas 8 percent achieve 100 percent completion. The distribution of participation rates for clinical screenings is similarly spread out (data not shown). The wide variation in participation rates may be due to differences in calculating participation rates—program administrators may consider every eligible employee a participant unless they actively

Figure 4.1: Employee Completion Rates of HRAs Among Employers That Offer HRAs

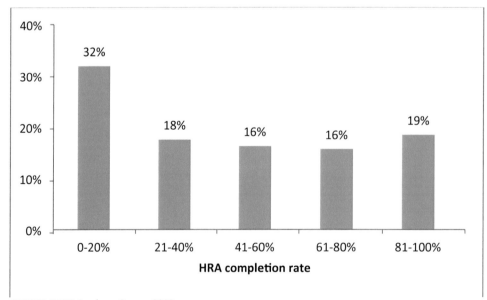

SOURCE: RAND Employer Survey, 2012.
NOTES: The graph represents information from employers with at least 50 employees that offer HRAs as a component of a wellness program. 51 percent of employers offer a wellness program, and 65 percent of those include an HRA.

opt out of the wellness program as opposed to considering only employees who actively enroll as participants (opt in). In many cases, participation rates are not tracked by the employer. One in six employers did not report participation rates for their wellness screening activities in the RAND employer survey. The role of incentives offered to encourage employees to complete the wellness screenings is discussed in Chapter 5.

Four of the five case study employers collect data on wellness program participation and outcomes. Employer B conducts annual employee wellness surveys to assess program participation, satisfaction, self-reported changes in behavior, and salient health concerns of the employees. Employer E collects data related only to program participation and wellness program contact with employees. Employers C and D are more sophisticated in terms of their data collection efforts and track data on both employee participation and health outcomes. Overall, program participation rates from our case studies are consistent with the rates documented in the CCA data. At Employer C, one-third of employees have participated in the quarterly biometrics screening program one or more times, and focus group participants reported that those screenings were the most visible and recognized component of the wellness program. Employer E, which does not offer incentives, reported that approximately 19 percent of the employee population completed a biometric screening.

Similarly, according to our analysis of the CCA data, HRA completion rates among the participating employers was comparable to the rates reported in our survey: The average rate for the four employers that contributed HRA data was 47 percent with a range from 14 to 61 percent (Figure 4.2).

4.1.2. Interventions

According to the RAND Employer Survey, participation in preventive *interventions* (i.e., lifestyle management and disease management programs) tends to be much lower than participation in wellness screenings (Figure 4.3). There is little variation in participation rates across employers for intervention programs, since most employers report low participation rates. The majority of employers (65 percent) have participation rates of 20 percent or less for disease management programs (Figure 4.4). This pattern holds true for all lifestyle management programs. For the smoking cessation and weight management programs, almost 90 percent of employers report participation rates of 20 percent or less. On average, employers in the RAND Employer Survey report that only 7 percent of their employees who smoke participated in smoking cessation programs in the past 12 months. The highest reported

Figure 4.2: Percentage of Employees That Completed an HRA in the CCA Analytic Sample

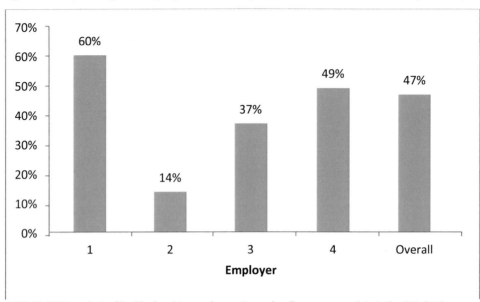

SOURCE: RAND analysis of health plan claims and screening and wellness program data in the CCA database.
NOTE: Data are shown for 2009 only.

Figure 4.3: Average Participation Rates of Employees Identified for Inclusion in Select Wellness Program Components

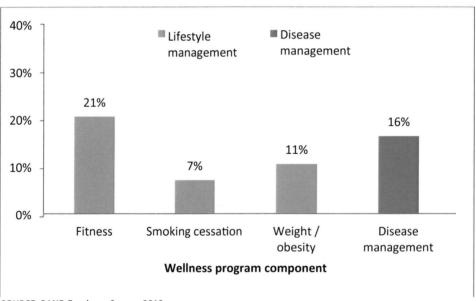

SOURCE: RAND Employer Survey, 2012.
NOTES: The graph represents information from employers with at least 50 employees that offer any lifestyle or disease management intervention as a component of a wellness program. 51 percent of employers offer a wellness program. Of those, 77 percent offer lifestyle management, and 56 percent offer disease management interventions. In most cases, eligibility to participate in lifestyle and disease management interventions are based on risk factors identified through screenings and health conditions identified through medical claims data. Rates reflect employees who were determined eligible for each program component.

Figure 4.4: Participation Rates of Employees Identified for Inclusion in Disease Management Among Employers with Any Disease Management Intervention

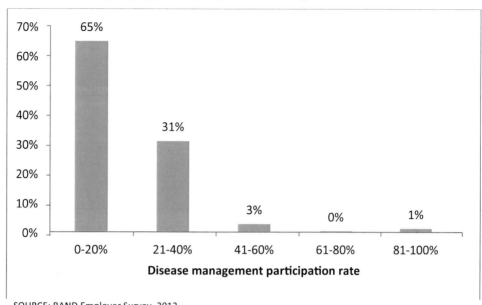

SOURCE: RAND Employer Survey, 2012.
NOTES: The graph represents information from employers with at least 50 employees that offer any disease management intervention as a component of a wellness program. 51 percent of employers offer a wellness program, and 56 percent of those offer a disease management intervention.

participation rate was 80 percent, but one in six employers (17 percent) reports no participation in this program at all. Fitness programs are the most well-attended intervention program, with an average uptake of 21 percent among targeted employees, but half of employers still report participation rates of 10 percent or less. Approximately two-fifths of employers did not report participation rates on the RAND employer survey for the intervention programs they offered.

At 55 percent, the overall lifestyle management participation rate among eligible employees in the CCA database was higher than that reported in the RAND Employer Survey (14 percent). If we exclude data from Employer 4, for which we could not distinguish between eligible and noneligible participants reliably and therefore could not estimate the participation rate,[19] the rate averages 36 percent (Figure 4.5).[20] These relatively high participation rates may partly be a consequence of the opt-out method that the program vendors use to calculate participation rates; that is, employees are regarded as participants

---

[19] The participation rate is calculated as the ratio of employees who are eligible for a program and chose to participate over all who are eligible. As some noneligible employees may participate in the program, the estimated rate at Employer 4 is likely to be biased upward.

[20] Participation rates based on the CCA data are not directly comparable to those from the RAND Employer Survey because of differences in included employers. Further, we determine participation rates based on an analysis of program data, whereas our survey results use employer-reported rates.

Figure 4.5: Participation Rates Among Employees Identified for Inclusion in Any Wellness Program Component in the CCA Analytic Sample

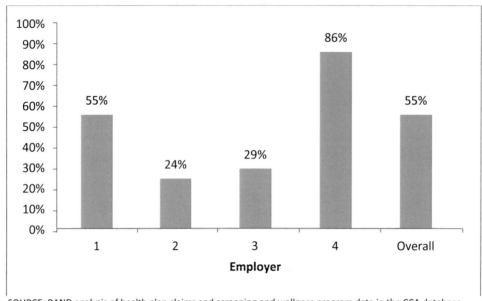

SOURCE: RAND analysis of health plan claims and screening and wellness program data in the CCA database.
NOTES: Data are shown for 2009 only. Employer 4 eligibility data were missing for all years; we assumed that all employees were eligible for the program(s) for which they had records.

unless they actively refuse to engage in the program. In opt-out programs, even one mailing of informational material counts as program participation. Conversely, other programs use an opt-in approach, under which only employees who actively enroll are considered participants.

We also analyzed the intensity of program engagement by calculating the unique number of program contacts per participating employee, either phone contacts or through mailing educational material to the employee. Phone contacts can be initiated by the program, referred to as "outbound calls," but are sometimes initiated by the employees, so called "inbound calls." The programs also offered a wide variety of online tools and resources but did not track their use at the employee level. Most employees had six contacts with the program (Figure 4.6), and about 20 percent of the overall contacts were by phone.

Two case study employers reported comparable participation rates. Approximately 41 percent of employees at Employer C participated in at least one health and wellness activity in the past five years, and 26 percent of employees use the onsite gym facilities. Annual employee surveys revealed that about half of all Employer B employees participated in worksite wellness activities. In 2010, approximately two-fifths of all participating employees did some type of activity at least twice a week. Individual

Figure 4.6: Average Number of Phone and Mail Contacts Received by Wellness Program Participants in the CCA Analytic Sample

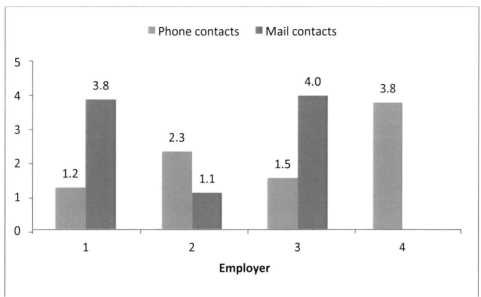

SOURCE: RAND analysis of health plan claims and screening and wellness program data in the CCA database.
NOTES: Data are shown for Employers 1–4 for 2009 only. Online contacts were not tracked at employee level. Employer 4 had data on phone contacts only.

walking, group walking challenges, and organized fitness classes were the most popular activities. More than a quarter of all employees participated in healthy eating wellness activities, such as the fruit and vegetable challenges.

Information that is available in the CCA database on the prevalence of risk factors among the four employers is shown in Figure 4.7. Overall, 28.1 percent of employees were obese, 40.0 percent were overweight, and high cholesterol was present in 7.4 percent of employees. Among the two employers in our sample with exercise data, 41.2 percent of employees did not get at least three days of exercise of at least 20 minutes per day, suggesting that many employees fell short of the DHHS physical activity guidelines of 150 minutes of exercise per week (Kolbe-Alexander et al., 2012). The prevalence of cigarette smoking was 15.9 percent for Employers 1 and 3 combined.

According to the CCA database, 38.1 percent of employees completing an HRA at Employers 1–4 were determined to be eligible for at least one wellness program (Figure 4.8). As we do not know the program eligibility criteria used for each employer, caution should be used in comparing proportions eligible across employers. Similarly, we cannot examine participation among eligibles by risk factor, as the proprietary criteria to determine program eligibility were not available to us.

Figure 4.7: Percentage of Employees with Selected Health Risk Among Those Who Completed an HRA

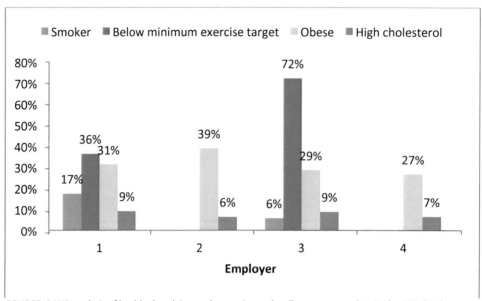

SOURCE: RAND analysis of health plan claims and screening and wellness program data in the CCA database.
NOTES: Smoking status and exercise data were not available for Employers 2 and 4. Smoking is defined as currently smoking cigarettes; target level of exercise is defined as at least 20 minutes of exercise per day on at least three days per week (Kolbe-Alexander et al., 2012); high cholesterol is defined as ≥ 240 mg/dL; obese is defined as BMI ≥ 30.

Figure 4.8: Percentage of Employees Who Were Identified for Inclusion in Any Wellness Program Among Those Who Completed an HRA in the CCA Analytic Sample

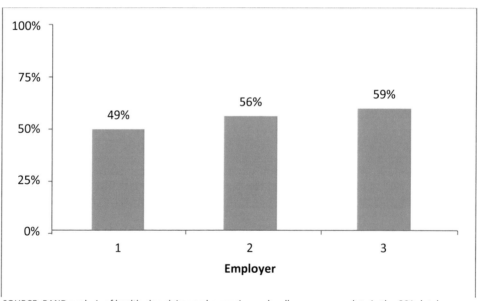

SOURCE: RAND analysis of health plan claims and screening and wellness program data in the CCA database.
NOTE: Only employers and employer years with complete eligibility data were used to generate the figure.

4.2. Effect on Health-Related Behaviors

To quantify the impact of wellness program participation on health-related behaviors, we examined differential changes between program participants and nonparticipants in exercise frequency and smoking status over time.

4.2.1. Exercise

We first examined the impact of program participation on exercise frequency. Our analysis was limited to the one employer with at least two years of data on exercise patterns available in the CCA database. At baseline, we estimate that 53 percent of its employees, who completed an HRA, met the recommended target of at least 150 minutes of exercise per week. We obtained this estimate by applying the median duration (45 minutes) of exercise defined as "vigorous physical activity" among adults aged 18–64 in the 2011 National Health Interview Survey [21](National Center for Health Statistics, 2012).

Figure 4.9: Percentage Distribution of Frequency of Exercise Among Employees in the CCA Analytic Sample Who Completed an HRA

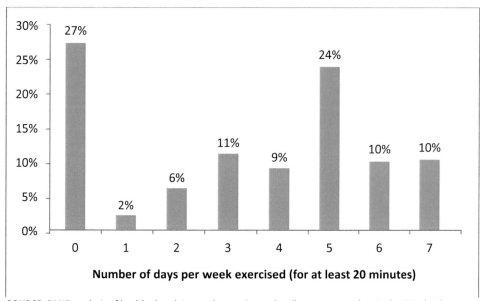

Number of days per week exercised (for at least 20 minutes)

SOURCE: RAND analysis of health plan claims and screening and wellness program data in the CCA database.
NOTES: Data are shown for Employer 1 for 2009 only. Exercise data were not available for analysis from Employers 2, 3, and 4.

---

[21] This estimate was obtained using 2011 National Health Interview Survey data for question ID AHB.100. The question asks adults aged 18 or older who report doing vigorous physician exercise: "About how long do you do these vigorous leisure-time physical activities each time?" We limited our analysis to adults aged 18 to 64 who responded to the question with a complete time duration value (N = 12,404).

The multivariate analysis of data from the CCA database, in which program participants are matched to similar nonparticipants at baseline, shows that participation in an exercise program is associated with a significant increase in exercise activities. The estimates show that current year participation is associated with 0.15 additional days of at least 20 minutes exercise per week in the same year and 0.11 days in the second year. But current-year program participation has no significant effect after the second year, as Figure 4.10 shows.[22]

The cumulative effects of exercise program participation are illustrated in Figure 4.11. We estimated that continuous participation in an exercise program over five years is associated with about 1.5 additional days of at least 20 minutes of exercise per week. Continuous participation in an exercise program requires strong motivation, and our results illustrate only the potential impact in a five-year period. Also, in the estimation of the program impacts, we were unable to fully control for unobserved residual differences between participants and nonparticipants, such as differential motivation. This is

Figure 4.10: Effect of Current-Year Exercise Program Participation on Exercise Frequency

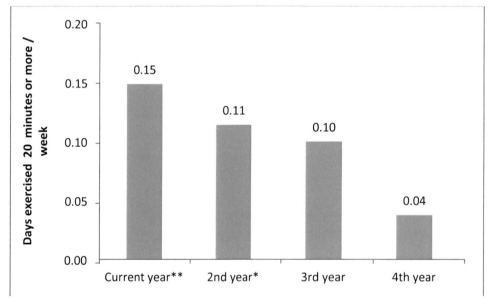

SOURCE: RAND analysis of health plan claims and screening and wellness program data in the CCA database.
NOTE: 2005–2010 data are from one employer; 2,303 propensity score matched pairs.
*p < 0.05; **p < 0.01.

---

[22] The analysis was based on the 2005–2010 data of one employer whose HRA contains self-reported exercise activities. The final analytical sample included 2,303 pairs successfully matched using propensity score.

45

Figure 4.11: Cumulative Simulated Effects of Exercise Program Participation on Exercise Frequency

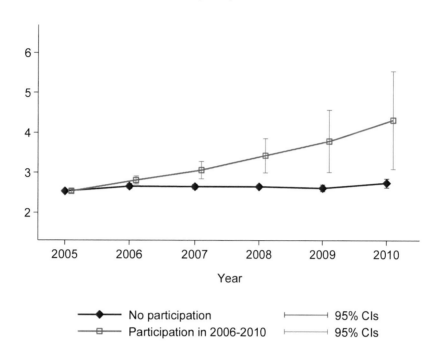

SOURCE: RAND analysis of health plan claims and screening and wellness program data in the CCA database.
NOTES: Simulation results are based on continuous participation in 2006–2010 of a population that has the average characteristics of the estimation sample; $p < 0.05$ for all years in 2006–2010. CI = confidence interval.

particularly a concern when some employees continuously participated in a program for five years, because these employees are more likely to be highly motivated.

4.2.2. Smoking

Next, we examined the impact of participation in a smoking cessation program on employees' ability to quit smoking. Our analysis was based on data for one employer with smoking data in the CCA database, for which 18 percent of employees reported at baseline that they smoked cigarettes. As illustrated in Figure 4.12, smoking rates decrease over time even among those smokers who did not participate in the smoking cessation program, but program participation is associated with a significantly larger reduction in smoking rates. One year of program participation decreases the smoking rate of participating smokers by nearly 30 percent in the first year compared to nonparticipating smokers. Program participation also has effects in the subsequent years, but the magnitude of the effect decreases over time, which becomes not statistically significant at the 5 percent confidence level in the fourth year.

46

Figure 4.12: Percentage of Smokers Who Continue Smoking After One-Year Participation in a Smoking Cessation Program, Compared to Nonparticipating Smokers

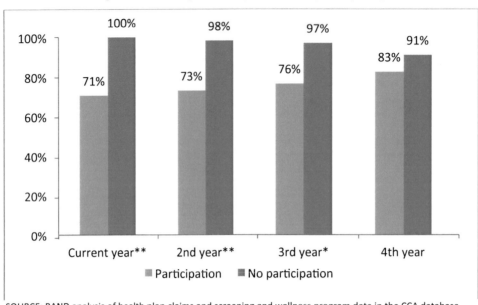

SOURCE: RAND analysis of health plan claims and screening and wellness program data in the CCA database.
NOTES: 2005–2010 data are from one employer; 746 propensity score matched pairs.
*p < 0.05; **p < 0.01.

Similarly, Employer D in the case studies stated that participation in a smoking cessation program helped 33 employees quit smoking between 2011 and 2012, which translated into a one percentage point reduction (from 32 percent to 31 percent) in the total number of tobacco users. Among the estimated 3,000 to 5,000 smokers employed by Employer B, participation in a wellness program helped 566 employees quit smoking and 695 employees reduce their tobacco use between 2006 and 2010. Neither employer had comparable data on employees who did not participate in the programs.

4.3. Effect on Health Status

In this section, we continue our analysis of program impacts by examining the consequence of program participation on body weight and cholesterol. Our analyses examine the immediate impacts and the impacts in subsequent years of program participation on these two health status measures. In addition, we simulated the cumulative effects if an employee participated in a program consecutively over a period of time.

4.3.1. Weight Control

The program impact on weight was analyzed for four employers in the CCA database. At baseline, 39 percent and 28 percent of employees were overweight and obese, respectively, across the four employers and only between 25 percent (Employer 1) and 38 percent (Employer 3) were of normal weight (Figure 4.13).

Our analysis of the CCA data shows that participation in a program aimed to control body weight, improve nutrition, or increase exercise is associated with a significant decrease in BMI. As shown in Figure 4.14, current-year participation in a weight control program is significantly associated with a reduction of BMI (kg/m^2) of about 0.15 in the same year, and the effect persists for two subsequent years. This change in the first three years corresponds to a weight loss of about 0.9 pound in an average woman of 165 pounds and 5 feet and 4 inches in height, or about one pound in an average man of 195 pounds and 5 feet and 9 inches in height (Figure 4.15).

As our simulation analysis shows, a typical employee, who continuously participates in a weight control program over five years, will have a reduction of 1.9 in BMI, whereas a comparable nonparticipant will

Figure 4.13: Percentage Distribution of BMI Categories Among Employees Who Completed an HRA

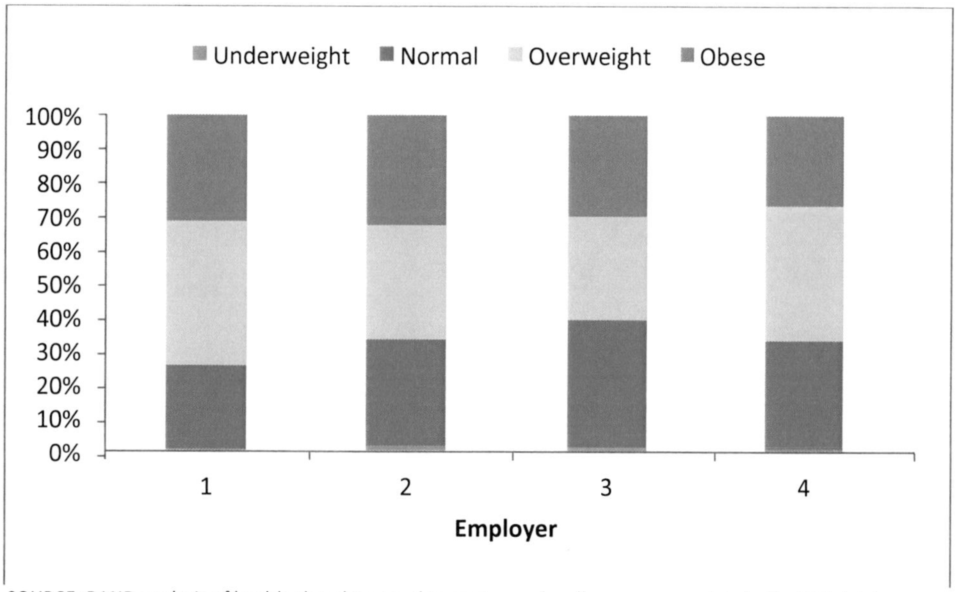

SOURCE: RAND analysis of health plan claims and screening and wellness program data in the CCA database (2009 data).
NOTE: Underweight, BMI < 18.5; normal, BMI ≥ 18.5 and < 25, overweight, BMI ≥ 25 and < 30, obese, BMI ≥ 30.

Figure 4.14: Effect of Current-Year Weight Control Program Participation on BMI

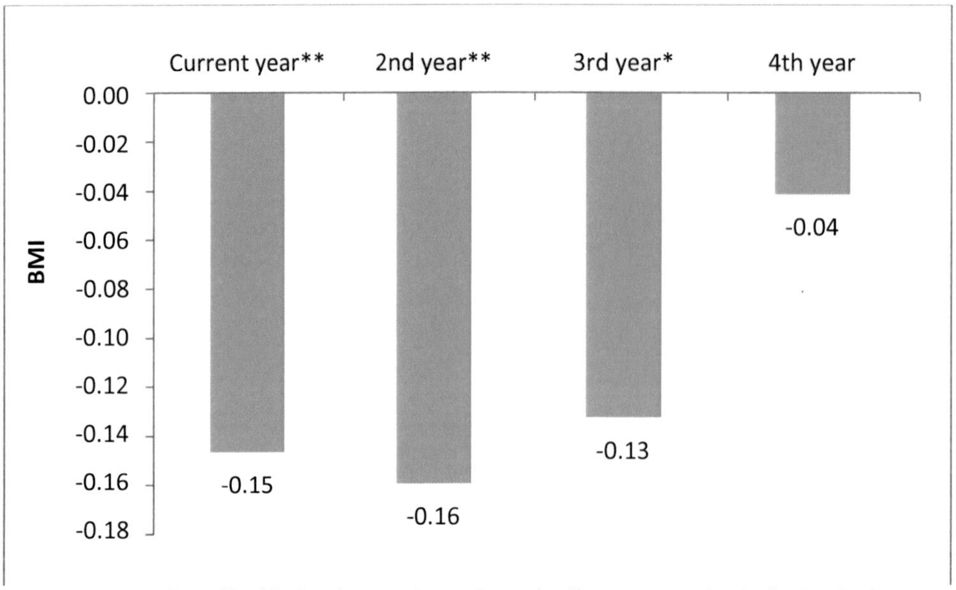

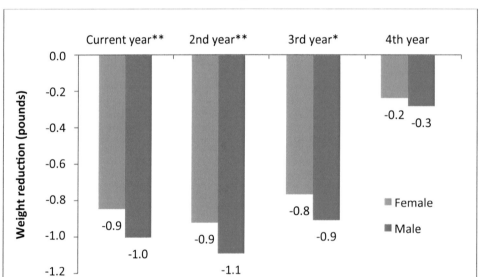

SOURCE: RAND analysis of health plan claims and screening and wellness program data in the CCA database.
NOTE: 2005–2010 data are from four employers; 3,924 propensity score matched pairs.
*p < 0.05; **p < 0.01.

Figure 4.15: Effect of Current Year Weight Control Program Participation on Body Weight in an Average Person

SOURCE: RAND analysis of health plan claims and screening and wellness program data in the CCA database.
NOTES: 2005–2010 data are from four employers; 3,924 propensity score matched pairs. According to CDC (2011), the average height and weight of an adult female are 63.8 inches and 164.7 pounds, respectively; the numbers for an adult male are 69.4 inches and 194.7 pounds, respectively. The BMI of an average adult (male or female) is 28.4.
*p < 0.05; **p < 0.01.

increase BMI by about 0.5. Figure 4.16 illustrates this effect, which corresponds to a relative weight loss (difference between two curves) of 10 pounds in an average woman of 165 pounds and 5 feet and 4 inches in height, or a weight loss of 13 pounds in an average man of 195 pounds and 5 feet and 9 inches in height.

We also simulated to what degree the program effect allows participants to transition from being obese to merely overweight and from being overweight to normal weight. Looking at program participants only, the simulations show that the proportion of overweight employee decreases slightly over time, whereas the share of obese employees decreases and more employees have normal weight (Figure 4.17). This pattern exists because obese employees do not achieve normal weight given the estimated program effects but rather go to being merely overweight. At the same time, a subset of overweight employees achieves normal weight. The combined effect is a mostly constant share of overweight employees but an increase in the number of normal weight employees at the expense of obese employees and a significant overall reduction in weight.

Figure 4.16: Cumulative Simulated Effects of Participation in a Weight Control Program on Body Weight over Five Years

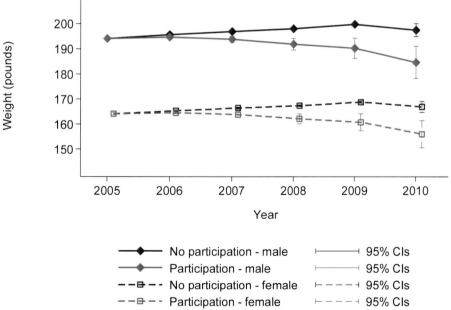

SOURCE: RAND analysis of health plan claims and screening and wellness program data in the CCA database.
NOTE: Simulation results are based on the continuous participation in 2006–2010 of an average woman or man in the United States; changes are significantly different at $p < 0.05$. CI = confidence interval.

Figure 4.17: Percentage Distribution of the Cumulative Simulated Effects of Consecutive Participation in a Weight Control Program on Employee Weight Status

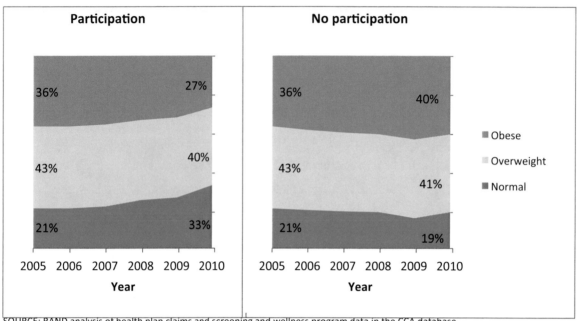

SOURCE: RAND analysis of health plan claims and screening and wellness program data in the CCA database.
NOTE: Simulation results are based on continuous participation in 2006–2010 of the model estimation sample.

In contrast, the proportion of obese employees among nonparticipants increases four percentage points and that of overweight and normal weight employees decreases slightly. This is because nonparticipants gain weight during the same time period. When comparing participants and nonparticipants, the relative difference becomes even more marked. Overall, we estimate that continuous participation in a weight loss program for over five years can be credited with a 13 percentage point decrease in obesity rates and a 14 percentage point increase in the share of normal weight employees, compared to nonparticipants.

Indeed, experiences of Employers B and C in the case studies support the results of our statistical analyses in that they show that employee participation in wellness activities has a positive short-term impact on a number of health behaviors, including eating habits and weight loss. Using employee surveys, Employer B identified that roughly half of all survey participants in 2010 reported positive changes in their walking activities and eating habits, whereas a quarter of participants reported getting closer to a healthy weight. One employee we interviewed also described the change in behaviors and attitudes that was attributed to participation in the wellness program: "People that never exercised, that were extremely overweight . . . you can see the difference in their lives, their activity levels, and weight loss. How when we have luncheons, no one is complaining that we don't have dessert or that we

51

have lots of salads and soup." Similarly, Employer C also found that its healthy eating and lifestyle management program, which offers educational information on nutrition and healthy eating, personalized phone support from health coaches, and online tracking to help participants monitor their eating patterns and health improvements, had a positive effect on health status. Of more than 100 individuals who completed the program, over 50 percent reduced their BMI, 92 percent reduced their blood pressure, 83 percent improved their blood sugar levels, and 100 percent improved cholesterol levels.

4.3.2. Cholesterol Control

We analyzed the program impact on cholesterol control for four employers in the CCA database. At baseline, 23 percent and 7 percent of employees had borderline and elevated blood cholesterol level, respectively, and around two-thirds of all employees had normal cholesterol levels (Figure 4.18.).

Wellness program participation was not associated with significant reductions in total cholesterol level, as Figure 4.19 illustrates. This lack of effect may be partly explained by the strong secular trend toward lower cholesterol levels that our simulation analysis shows (Figure 4.20).

Figure 4.18: Percentage Distribution of Total Cholesterol Levels Among Employees Who Completed an HRA

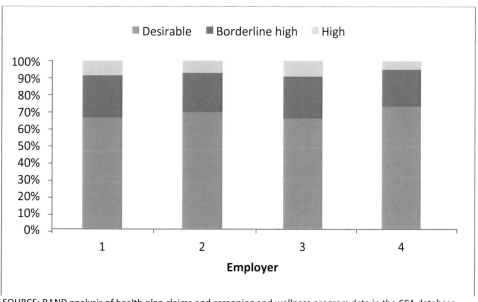

SOURCE: RAND analysis of health plan claims and screening and wellness program data in the CCA database (2009 data).
NOTES: Normal total blood cholesterol, < 200 mg/dl; borderline high, ≥ 200 mg/dl and < 240; high, ≥ 240 mg/dl. Total cholesterol was used as the outcome of interest, because data for total cholesterol rather than low-density lipoprotein cholesterol, was complete for a much larger proportion of employees.

Figure 4.19: Effect of One-Year Participation in a Cholesterol Program on Total Cholesterol Level

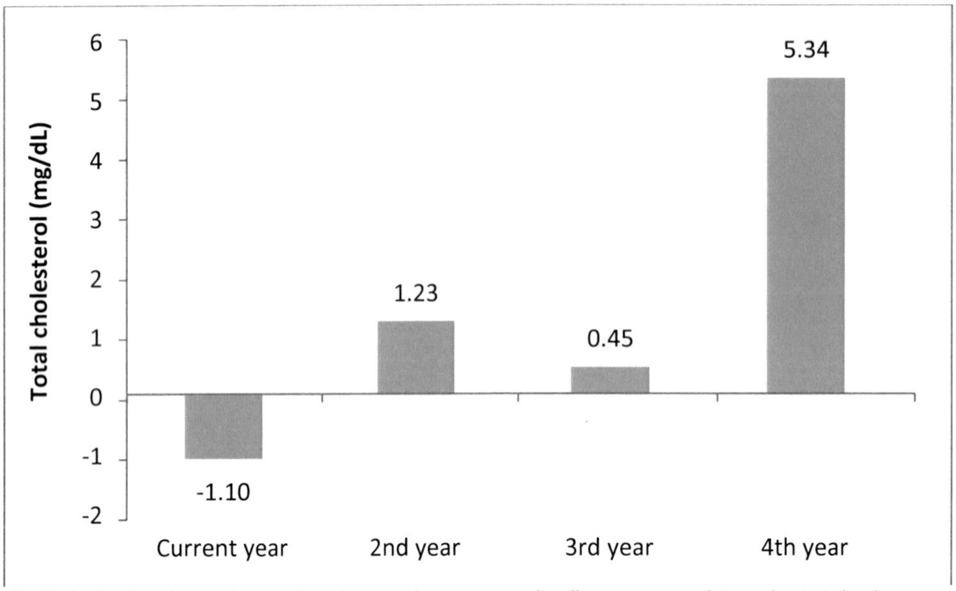

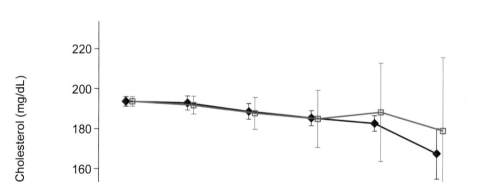

SOURCE: RAND analysis of health plan claims and screening and wellness program data in the CCA database.
NOTE: 2005–2010 data are from four employers; 1,341 propensity score matched pairs.
*p < 0.05; **p. < 0.01.

Figure 4.20: Cumulative Simulated Effects of Cholesterol Program Participation on Cholesterol Levels

SOURCE: RAND analysis of health plan claims and screening and wellness program data in the CCA database.
NOTE: Simulation results are based on continuous participation in 2006–2010 of a population that has the average characteristics of the estimation sample; p > 0.05 for all years in 2006–2010. CI = confidence interval.

Nonetheless, a trend analysis of data from Employer C in the case studies found that individuals who participated in its biometrics screening program and had at least two follow-up screenings showed improvements on a variety of biometric outcomes, including cholesterol levels. Results indicate that approximately 65 percent improved cholesterol levels, 70 percent of participants lost weight, and 80 percent of individuals with hypertension lowered their blood pressure.

4.4. Effect on Health Care Cost and Utilization

4.4.1. Perceived Cost Savings

Data from the RAND Employer Survey suggest that employers view the impact of their wellness programs overwhelmingly as positive (Figure 4.21). More than 60 percent stated that their program reduced health care cost, and around four-fifths reported that it decreased absenteeism and increased productivity. But less than half of the employers (44 percent) reported regularly evaluating their wellness programs, and only 2 percent provided actual savings estimates.

Case study findings also suggest that employers perceive programs as improving affordability of coverage, even though four of the five case study employers have not yet formally evaluated the program's impact on health care cost or return on investment, because of lack of access to data, limited capabilities and methodological questions. Results of a study conducted at

Figure 4.21: Percentage of Employers Reporting Benefits from Their Wellness Program

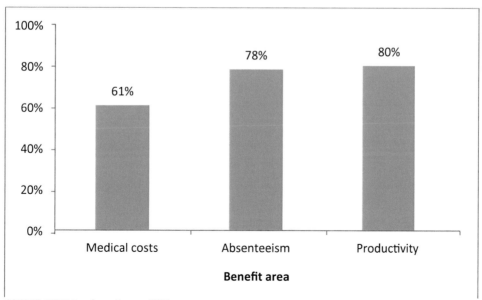

SOURCE: RAND Employer Survey, 2012.
NOTE: The graph represents information from the subset of employers with at least 50 employees that offer a wellness program (51 percent).

54

Employer E support the importance of verifying program impact. When Employer E conducted an evaluation of its fitness leave benefit, which provides paid leave time of up to three hours a week for fitness activities, it found that every 20 hours of fitness leave was associated with only a one hour reduction in sick leave.

Employer C's health plan evaluated savings derived from the wellness program by comparing the employer's health care cost trend against an industry benchmark. The evaluation showed that the employer saved $111 per member in 2009 and $261 in 2010. Managers at Employer C shared that the wellness programs constitute an investment of less than 1 percent of their total health care costs but has reduced medical expenses by approximately two to three percentage points below industry trend since 2009. Although leaders were not able to pinpoint the exact sources of the savings, they noted that savings align with measurable changes in care utilization patterns: "We noticed the savings since we've begun wellness initiatives . . . our emergency room visits have gone down, and we are above benchmark for all preventive care screenings."

Employer A commissioned a study to inform its program evaluation strategy in the same way that other organizations measure the impact of their wellness programs. The study recommended focusing on measuring program participation and satisfaction through surveys of participants and nonparticipants. Organizational leaders at Employer A explained that researchers who led the evaluation recommended tracking selected outcome metrics, such as absenteeism and satisfaction, rather than ROI because "many experts even question whether you should look at ROI." Absenteeism was the only metric that the researchers felt was measurable and useful for Employer A's ROI analysis. Productivity was deemed impossible to measure given the nature of labor at the organization, whereas health outcomes were ruled out because of privacy concerns. Privacy issues can become a hurdle "because it's difficult to get people to give up personal information about their weight and health issues."

4.4.2. Evidence for Cost Savings

We estimated the impact of wellness program participation using the CCA data. Figure 4.22 displays unadjusted trends in medical costs for the four employers included in the analytic sample for this analysis.

Figure 4.22: Trends in Health Care Costs per Health Plan Member per Month Among Employers in the CCA Analytic Sample

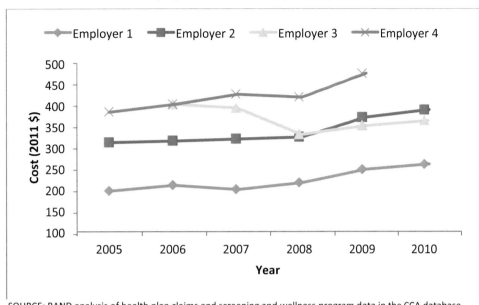

SOURCE: RAND analysis of health plan claims and screening and wellness program data in the CCA database.
NOTES: PMPM data are not available for Employer 3 in 2005 and Employer 4 in 2010. Costs are adjusted to 2011 dollars using the Consumer Price Index (annual average, CPI, all urban consumers, U.S. city average, all items).

Figure 4.23 shows our analysis of the association between wellness program participation and overall health care cost for employers in the CCA database. Program participation is associated with a trend toward lower health care costs, but the changes are not statistically significant. We estimate that program participation is associated with a reduction of $2.38 PMPM in the first year and that the effect increases to up to $11.12 PMPM in the fourth year, both nonsignificant changes (Figure 4.23). This change roughly corresponds to a 0.5 percent and 2.5 percent decrease in cost of coverage,[23] respectively. A power calculation shows that we would have been able to statistically detect a difference of $31.50 in PMPM cost, almost three times the actually observed point estimate.

Figure 4.24 shows the results of our simulation analysis, which compares trends in overall health care cost of program participants and nonparticipants over five years. The graph illustrates the nonstatistically significant trend toward lower health care cost of program participants. Over a five-year period, the cumulative difference between the two groups is $65.50 per member per month, implying average annual cost reductions of $157.

---

[23] According KFF/HRET (2011), "The average premium for single coverage in 2011 is $452 per month or $5,429 per year." (KFF/HRET, 2011) We used 2011 insurance premiums, as the medical costs in the analysis were adjusted to the 2011 U.S. dollars.

Figure 4.23: Effect of One-Year Wellness Program Participation on Total Health Care Costs per Health Plan Member per Month

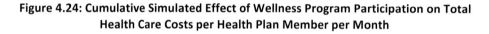

SOURCE: RAND analysis of health plan claims and screening and wellness program data in the CCA database.
NOTE: 2005–2010 data are from four employers; 12,127 propensity score matched pairs.
*p < 0.05; **p < 0.01.

Figure 4.24: Cumulative Simulated Effect of Wellness Program Participation on Total Health Care Costs per Health Plan Member per Month

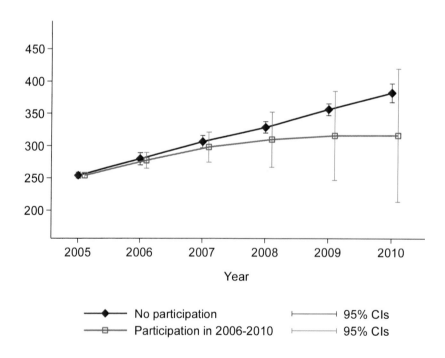

SOURCE: RAND analysis of health plan claims and screening and wellness program data in the CCA database.
NOTE: Simulation results are based on continuous participation in 2006–2010 of a population that has the average characteristics of the estimation sample; p > 0.05 for all years in 2006–2010. CI = confidence interval.

We decomposed the simulated trends in total PMPM cost, and the results suggest that the trends are primarily driven by the reduction in inpatient cost, accounting for nearly two-thirds of the total cost reduction. Reductions in outpatient costs and prescription drug cost account for 28 percent and 10 percent, respectively (Figure 4.25). Corresponding to these cost reduction trends are declines in inpatient admissions and emergency department visits. During the same time period, inpatient admissions and emergency department visits reduce by 22 and 42 per 1,000 employee years, respectively (Figures 4.26 and 4.27). In contrast, inpatient admissions and emergency department visits among the comparison group either increase or slightly decrease. However, note that all estimates are not statistically significant at the 5 percent confidence level.

4.5. Discussion of the Evidence on impact

4.5.1. Program Uptake

The RAND Employer Survey data show that, on average, about half of employees at employers with wellness programs undergo clinical screening and/or complete an HRA but also that variation across employers is substantial, and a large proportion of employers do not track participation rates. As ascertaining health risks at the individual level is critical to create awareness and direct employers to

Figure 4.25: Percentage Distribution of Cumulative Cost Savings per Member per Month After Five Years of Participation in a Wellness Program, by Type of Health Care Services

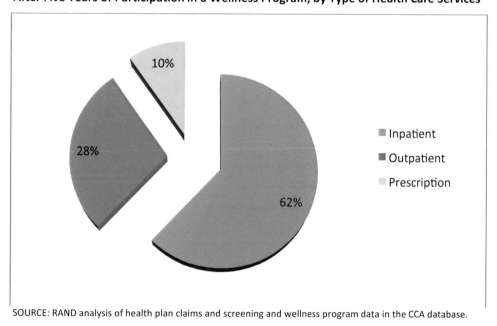

SOURCE: RAND analysis of health plan claims and screening and wellness program data in the CCA database.

58

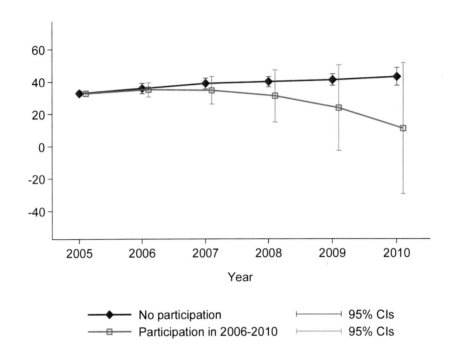

Figure 4.26: Cumulative Simulated Effects of Wellness Program Participation on Inpatient Admissions

No participation — 95% CIs
Participation in 2006-2010 — 95% CIs

SOURCE: RAND analysis of health plan claims and screening and wellness program data in the CCA database.
NOTE: Simulation results are based on continuous participation in 2006–2010 of a population that has the average characteristics of the estimation sample; p > 0.05 for all years in 2006–2010. CI = confidence interval.

appropriate resources and programs, low uptake of wellness screening activities will limit program impact. In addition, tracking employer-level health risk data is invaluable to assess program impact and prioritize interventions.

Similarly, from RAND's Employer Survey, we find that participation rates in interventions under wellness programs are even lower, ranging between 7 and 21 percent, depending on program target, and again with substantial variation. The CCA data analysis shows similar rates of HRA completion, as nearly half of employees completed an HRA, but higher participation rates in lifestyle management programs, with an average uptake of about one-third and a range from 24 percent to 55 percent participation rate. This overall limited uptake will impede the ability of employers to realize the full value of their investment in workplace wellness (Goetzel et al., 2007).

Figure 4.27: Cumulative Simulated Effects of Wellness Program Participation on Emergency Department Visits

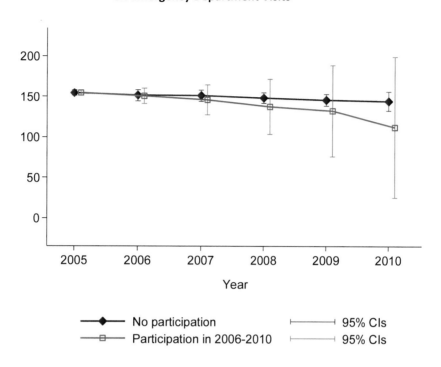

SOURCE: RAND analysis of health plan claims and screening and wellness program data in the CCA database.
NOTE: Simulation results are based on continuous participation in 2006–2010 of a population that has the average characteristics of the estimation sample; p > 0.05 for all years in 2006–2010. CI = confidence interval.

Findings from our case studies corroborate our survey results of limited and variable uptake. Participation in clinical screenings ranged from 19 percent to 100 percent among employers, though full participation was achieved in one case study employer only after it introduced a $50 weekly insurance premium surcharge on those employees who did not undergo biometric screening. Wellness intervention uptake rates varied based on the nature of the intervention and on how uptake was defined   For example, although one employer reported that 41 percent of employees had participated in at least one activity in the past five years, another employer claimed that half of employees annually participated in a wellness activity.

Focus group participants indicate that poor accessibility to wellness activities because of rigid work schedules and wait times can limit wellness benefits. Employer E, which employs both maintenance and office workers, provides employees with paid time off work to participate in wellness activities, such as using the gym or participating in classes. White collar employees took advantage of this benefit, whereas access for maintenance workers was commonly limited by work schedules and mandatory overtime. Similarly, focus group participants at Employer C mentioned that they mostly have flexible work schedules, but long and often unpredictable wait times for onsite clinical screenings were a "nuisance" and discouraged their participation. (Chapter 6 describes barriers to program uptake in detail.)

Although not nationally representative, other industry surveys have painted a picture that is consistent with our results. For example, in a 2010 nonrepresentative survey of employers, HRA and clinical screening rates over 50 percent were achieved by only about a third and a sixth of organizations, respectively (Nyce, 2010). Participation rates were much lower for individualized interventions, such as weight management and health coaching. The level of participation is difficult to quantify precisely, because between 35 and 40 percent of employers were not aware of the actual participation rates for many activities (Nyce, 2010). Surveys of individual employees rather than employers tell a similar story. A 2010 nonrepresentative survey of employees by Hewitt Associates (now Aon Hewitt) and the National Business Group on Health suggests that clinical screenings are the wellness activity with the highest participation rate, at 61 percent. The same survey indicates that 41 percent of workers reported completing an HRA. More than half of the workers who were offered an HRA but did not complete it believed that their employer did not offer one (National Business Group on Health, 2010). A recent three-year evaluation of the Blue Cross Blue Shield's comprehensive wellness program in 15 employer groups showed an HRA completion rate of 44 percent and program participation rates between 14 and 97 percent (Hochart and Lang, 2011).

4.5.2. Impact on Health-Related Behaviors and Health Outcomes

Our analyses of individual program participation data from the CCA provide evidence for program effectiveness in a small sample of employers. We find statistically significant and meaningful improvements in exercise frequency, smoking behavior, and weight control. Those improvements are sustainable over an observation period of four years, and our simulation analyses point to cumulative effects with ongoing program participation. Note that our results on health behaviors are based on single employer analyses because of data availability, but those on health outcomes are based on four employers. To illustrate the program effectiveness, comparing to nonparticipants shows that continuous participation in a weight control program for five years would result in a relative weight loss of 10 pounds in an average woman or 13 pounds in an average man. The only exception in our data was cholesterol control, which was not significantly better in program participants compared to nonparticipants. This lack of impact may be explained by a strong downward trend in cholesterol levels in the population. This positive assessment was echoed by the employers in our case studies, but it should be qualified that they did not evaluate program impact rigorously and sometimes based their assessment on employee testimonials.

Our review of the published literature shows consistent results (Osilla et al., 2012). We identified 13 studies that evaluated program impact on exercise patterns, of which eight (62 percent) found improvements in physical activity (Gold, Anderson and Serxner, 2000; Nichols et al., 2000; Campbell et al., 2002; Purath et al., 2004; Herman et al., 2006; Goetzel et al., 2007; Faghri et al., 2008; MacKinnon et al., 2010). Six of 12 studies that used diet as an outcome reported significant improvement, including higher fruit and vegetable consumption and lower fat and energy intake (Gold, Anderson and Serxner, 2000; Ozminkowski et al., 2000; Campbell et al., 2002; Cook et al., 2007; French et al., 2010; MacKinnon et al., 2010).

Published research also suggests that workplace wellness programs can improve health status, as measured with physiological markers, such as BMI, cholesterol levels, and blood pressure. Six studies found beneficial effects in one or more outcomes, including BMI or weight (Ozminkowski et al., 2000; Herman et al., 2006; Racette et al., 2009; MacKinnon et al., 2010; Siegel et al., 2010; Barham et al., 2011), diastolic blood pressure (Ozminkowski et al., 2000), and body fat (Racette et al., 2009).

A more recent randomized controlled trial that compared two types of health promotion programs (a less interactive and a more interactive program) to a hobby-oriented comparison group found that both intervention groups had improvements in consumer activation (e.g., improved attitudes, knowledge, and behaviors about health), and that the more interactive intervention improved health risks more than the less interaction intervention. Those effects were sustainable over two years (Terry et al., 2011).

There is some evidence that smoking cessation programs have positive effects on reducing or stopping tobacco use in the short term. One systematic review found that workplace interventions promoting smoking cessation, such as group and individual counseling, as well as nicotine replacement therapy increased smoking cessation rates compared to the control group (Cahill, Moher and Lancaster, 2008). Another found higher quit rates among participants than nonparticipants in smoking cessation programs in the majority of studies (85 percent), even after one-year follow-up (Osilla et al., 2012). Two systematic reviews concluded that smoking cessation programs accompanied by consumer incentives and/or workplace competitions resulted in a reduction in self-reported tobacco use and higher quit rates (Leeks et al., 2010; Cahill and Perera, 2011). However, Cahill, Moher, and Lancaster (2008) report that these behavior changes were not sustainable beyond 12 months.

4.5.3. Impact on Health Care Cost and Utilization

In the RAND Employer Survey, employers overwhelmingly expressed confidence that workplace wellness programs help employers to reduce their medical cost, absenteeism, and health-related productivity losses. But at the same time, only about half stated that they have evaluated program impact formally and only 2 percent reported estimating actual savings. Similarly, none of our five case study employers had conducted a formal evaluation of their programs on cost; only one employer had requested an assessment of cost impact from its health plan.

Predominately positive reports in the published literature may have contributed to this optimistic view. A widely referenced meta-analysis by Baicker, Cutler, and Song (2010) reported that the average return on investment for wellness programs was about $3 for every dollar invested for both medical cost and cost of absenteeism. Average savings in medical costs were $358 per year with a range of $426 increased spending to $1,168 savings. When considering only randomized controlled trials, the savings estimates were more narrowly bounded between $11 and $626 per year (Baicker, Cutler and Song, 2010). Our own systematic review for this project (Osilla et al., 2012) (Osilla et al., 2012) identified eight studies on the effect of wellness programs on health care costs, and all except one found significant decreases (Aldana et al., 2005). Effects of these programs included a reduction in direct medical costs ranging from $176 to $1,539 per participant per year (Naydeck et al., 2008; Milani and Lavie, 2009; Henke et al., 2011). An evaluation of the Johnson & Johnson worksite health promotion program for 2002 to 2008 estimated $565 annual savings per employee (Henke et al., 2011).

But not all wellness program evaluations find cost reductions. Liu et al. (2012) published an evaluation of PepsiCo's health and wellness program and found that disease management but not lifestyle management interventions were associated with lower health care cost after three years.(Liu et al., 2012) The same pattern was observed by Nyman et al. (2010), who looked at the University of Minnesota's care management programs. The authors concluded that overall savings were lower than the program cost. The Blue Cross Blue Shield of Kansas City's wellness program found an increase in medical cost of about $600 per employee per year among participating employers. However, those estimates were not adjusted for employee risk and demographic characteristics (Hochart and Lang, 2011).

Our analysis of the CCA data points to a lower cost trend in program participants compared to nonparticipants, but the overall difference on overall health care cost is not statistically significant year-on-year or in the simulation of the cumulative effect over five years (Nyman, Barleen and Abraham, 2010). But it is noteworthy that our results indicate that use of inpatient and emergency department care decreased among participants.

Differences between our and published estimates of the effect of wellness programs on health care cost may be partly due to different analytic designs. Our approach yields a narrowly defined estimate of the effect of a lifestyle management program, because we compare participants to nonparticipants. Other evaluations that compare across employers can also capture employer-level differences, such as in benefit design and wellness culture, and the presence of other programs, such as disease management interventions.

4.5.4. Limitations

As with all observational designs, it is possible that results may suffer from bias, but any residual bias is likely to be small. First, we used propensity score matching to account for observable differences between nonparticipants and participants, such as age, sex, comorbidities, and prior health care use. Second, our approach adjusted for unobservable differences that are constant over time, such as an individual's motivation to improve health-related behavior. Thus, one would have to assume unobservable characteristics that vary over time and are associated with our endpoints to attribute our estimates to bias.

Our statistical analysis is based on a small number of large employers, who contracted with a national vendor to implement wellness programs. Those programs are likely to be highly sophisticated and professionally executed, and their results may not be generalizable to other programs that operate with fewer resources.

64

In spite of the large starting sample, our effective sample size remains small, because of limited program uptake, and even a five-year follow-up period may not have been long enough to detect cost changes, because of the long latency period for health-related behaviors to affect health care cost. However, our calculations confirm that the study was adequately powered to detect a meaningful change in health care cost (i.e., a $378 reduction in annual health care cost per employee), which is well within the range of previously published estimates.

We did not have access to program fees, as they are considered proprietary information by the wellness program vendors, and cannot estimate the net impact of the programs on cost of coverage. As a reference point, the above-referenced meta-analysis of Baicker, Cutler, and Song (2010) reported an average annual program cost of $144 per employee, which would be slightly less than our average annual savings estimate of $157 by the fifth program year.

Last, there may be beneficial program effects on outcomes that could not be measured using the available data, such as absenteeism, productivity, employee morale, workforce retention, and workplace culture.

4.5.5. Conclusion

To our knowledge, our study is the largest evaluation of lifestyle management programs to date. Consistent with published evidence, we find solid evidence that well-run programs operated by committed employers can meaningfully improve the health-related behaviors and health status of participating employees.

It is not clear at this point whether improved health-related behavior will translate into lower health care cost, but there is reason to be optimistic: We find decreases, albeit not statistically significant, in hospital and emergency department use, which are important cost drivers. The sustainable improvements in health status ought to translate into a lower rate of chronic disease and thus long-term reductions in health care cost. But the effect size of lifestyle management may not be as large as previously estimated. Our estimates point to savings, after five years, that are, with statistical confidence, below $378 per employee per year or about 7 percent of cost of coverage (Mercer, 2010). In other words, participation in lifestyle management interventions is associated with a reduction in direct medical costs of below 7 percent among participants. The effect on overall costs of coverage at the employer level will then depend on the share of employees participating in such programs and on program fees.

Chapter 5: The Role of Incentives

This chapter begins by summarizing the laws and regulations pertaining to the use of financial incentives for wellness programs. Evidence from the RAND Employer Survey and the CCA database and findings from case study employers are then used to describe the prevalence of incentives, common types of incentives such as cash rewards, novelty items and health care premium differentials, and their role in increasing participation rates or achieving better health outcomes.

5.1. Background

Employers have a strong interest in the use of incentives to encourage participation in workplace wellness programs, because of low participation rates and evidence suggesting that incentives can encourage healthy lifestyles (James, 2012). Evidence from the peer-reviewed literature suggests that targeted incentives can help to influence behaviors in the short term and increase participation in wellness programs (Volpp, 2009; Osilla et al., 2012). As limited program engagement continues to be seen as a key obstacle to success, employers and program vendors have eagerly responded to this emerging evidence by building rewards into their offerings.

5.2. Regulation on the Use of Incentives in Workplace Wellness Programs

A number of laws and regulations at the federal and state levels impose limits on the use of financial incentives in certain types of wellness programs. In general, state insurance regulations and federal regulations under the Public Health Service Act, the Employee Retirement Income Security Act (ERISA), and the tax code affect incentives offered through insured group health plans. Self-insured group health plans are generally exempt from state insurance regulations but remain subject to federal regulation. Mello and Rosenthal recently provided an overview focusing on the federal statutes. (Mello and Rosenthal, 2008) Incentives offered by an employer outside the context of a group health plan may still be subject to state or federal laws and regulations.

Before passage of the Affordable Care Act, the most significant applicable federal requirements were the HIPAA nondiscrimination provisions. In addition to HIPAA, other federal laws, such as GINA and the ADA, may apply to certain wellness programs. Under the HIPAA nondiscrimination rules, an individual cannot be denied eligibility or continued eligibility for benefits or charged more for group health coverage based on any health factor. However, an exception allows plans to offer incentives in the context of a wellness program that meets certain requirements. If none of the conditions for obtaining a reward under a wellness program is based on an individual satisfying a standard related to a health factor and participation in the program is made available to all similarly situated individuals, then, generally, the program will be outside the scope of the nondiscrimination requirements. Current law states that wellness programs that condition a reward on an individual satisfying a standard related to a health factor must meet the following requirements to be permissible under the HIPAA nondiscrimination rules (U.S. Department of Labor).

(1) The total reward for all the plan's wellness programs that require satisfaction of a standard related to a health factor must not exceed 20 percent of the cost of employee-only coverage under the plan. If dependents (such as spouses and/or dependent children) may participate in the wellness program, the reward must not exceed 20 percent of the cost of the coverage in which an employee and any dependents are enrolled.

(2) The program must be reasonably designed to promote health and prevent disease.

(3) The program must give individuals eligible to participate the opportunity to qualify for the reward at least once per year.

(4) The reward must be available to all similarly situated individuals. by providing The program must allow a reasonable alternative standard (or waiver of the initial standard) for obtaining the reward to any individual for whom it is unreasonably difficult because of a medical condition, or medically inadvisable, to satisfy the initial standard.

(5) The plan must disclose in all materials describing the terms of the program and the availability of a reasonable alternative standard (or the possibility of a waiver of the initial standard).

The Affordable Care Act substantially adopted the requirements of the existing HIPAA nondiscrimination regulations, with some changes. It raises the allowable value of incentives from 20 percent to 30 percent of the cost of coverage in 2014 and provides discretion to the Secretaries of Labor, Health and Human Services, and the Treasury to increase the reward to up to 50 percent of the cost of coverage if they determine that such an increase is appropriate. In addition, final wellness program rules implementing these provisions of the ACA would allow employers to charge tobacco users up to 50 percent more in premiums than nonusers, if they also provide a tobacco cessation wellness program (consistent with section 2705(j) of the Public Health Service Act), that would eliminate the surcharge for participants (*Federal Register,* 2012).

Other federal laws impose restrictions on incentives for health standard attainment under wellness programs irrespective of whether they are offered under an employer's group health plan or outside this plan (i.e., directly by the employer). The ADA states that individuals with health conditions that qualify as a disability under ADA must not be penalized (or have a reward withheld) on the basis of their disability. Certain conditions, such as severe obesity, may qualify as a disability, which would limit an employer's ability to offer incentives for weight loss (U.S. Department of Health and Human Services, 2004).

In contrast to the restrictions on incentives for attaining health-related standards, rewards related only to program participation or completion of HRAs (which do not require individuals to meet a health-related factor) is largely permissible under federal law. Some restrictions exist on the scope of data collection from HRAs. The ADA largely prohibits the employer from collecting information about disabilities but allows questions on lifestyles and disabilities on HRAs as long as participation is voluntary and information is not used to discriminate and is kept separate from employment records (Mastroianni, 2009). Similarly, strong financial incentives could be interpreted by the courts as violating the ADA requirement of voluntary data provision (Mello and Rosenthal, 2008).

In addition, GINA prohibits employers from collecting genetic information (which includes family medical history) for underwriting purposes (which includes such rewards as a premium discount for completing an HRA). Thus, wellness incentives can be offered only for completion of an HRA that contains questions about family medical history if answers to those particular questions are not required to receive the incentive. Although experts disagree on the value of this information to wellness programs, some suggest that the practical impact has been the elimination of these questions from most HRAs (Tu and Mayrell, 2010).

A number of other federal laws and regulations might affect incentives under workplace wellness programs, although all potential ramifications are unclear and would ultimately be determined through the courts. These statutes include provisions of ERISA, in addition to the HIPAA nondiscrimination and GINA rules, the Consolidated Omnibus Budget Reconciliation Act (COBRA), and federal civil rights and privacy laws, including the ADA and various aspects of the tax code (Mello and Rosenthal, 2008).

The HIPAA nondiscrimination rules and the Affordable Care Act market reforms regarding wellness programs provide a federal floor. State laws and regulations must be at least as protective as the federal requirements but may be more protective. Most states have nondiscrimination laws applicable to insured group health plans that limit the use of incentives for wellness programs. These regulations generally limit the types of information that can be used as the basis for charging different premiums for different employees. A number of states have passed laws that mirror the HIPAA nondiscrimination rules and include the exception to allow for incentives within the context of wellness programs that meet certain requirements. These rules facilitate the use of wellness program incentives by group health plans and align with the requirements of the final rules under the Affordable Care Act. Many states have passed laws that prohibit employers from penalizing workers for legal activities outside work, with some laws specifically protecting off-the-job tobacco use. Civil rights laws, including privacy protections, may restrict what information an employer can collect or what tests they can impose on employees on a nonvoluntary basis. In one frequently cited example, the Massachusetts Supreme Court ruled against lawn-care company Scotts, finding that the termination of an employee based on a positive biometric screening for nicotine was illegal. The employee had never smoked on the job, and although Massachusetts did not have a statute in place specifically protecting legal behavior outside work, the court ruled that the drug screen constituted an unreasonable search and had violated the employee's right to privacy.

The trade literature and our experts suggest that employers are cautious in expanding incentives to reward wellness program results, because of real and perceived legal restrictions under the different applicable statutes. Employers view incentives for health standard attainment as an area with substantial compliance risk and therefore may be less likely to use incentives to reward results rather than program participation.

5.3. Current Prevalence of Use of Incentives

The RAND Employer Survey results indicate that nationally, of the 51 percent of employers who offer workplace wellness programs, over two-thirds (69 percent) use financial incentives as a strategy to encourage employees to use wellness programs. Incentives for HRA completion and lifestyle management programs are most common and are offered by about 30 percent of employers with a wellness program. Although incentives are provided for clinical screenings that may identify chronic conditions targeted through disease management, incentives for participation in disease management are offered by only a few employers (4 percent), as Figure 5.1 shows.

The majority (90 percent) of employers that do not use incentives did not indicate any intent to introduce them in the next two years. However, between 20 and 30 percent of employers with incentives currently plan to start offering additional incentives for participation, completion, and health results, and 15 percent indicated an interest in increasing the amount of incentives for program participation.

Similarly, four of the five employers in our case studies used some type of financial incentives to promote wellness program participation and/or behavior change (Table 5.1). Incentives were triggered for completing a biometric screening (Employers B,[24] C, and D) or an HRA (Employer C). Four employers (Employers A, B, C, and D) used incentives to encourage employees to quit smoking, although only one required that employees verify their smoking status through a blood test (Employer D). Employer E

Figure 5.1: Percentage of Employers That Use Monetary Incentives for Participation Among Employers That Offer Wellness Programs

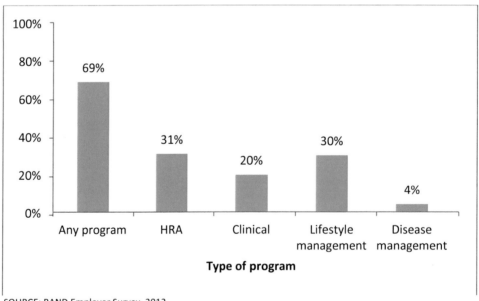

SOURCE: RAND Employer Survey, 2012.
NOTES: The graph represents information from the subset of employers with at least 50 employees that offer a wellness program (51 percent). Among those, 65 percent have an HRA, 49 percent have clinical screenings, 77 percent offer lifestyle management, and 56 percent offer disease management interventions.

---

[24] Employer B piloted an incentive of reduced copayments to participate in a health screening at one site.

Table 5.1: Incentives Offered by Case Study Employers

Case Study Employers	Annual Financial Incentives
Employer A	**Smoking:** $50 annual insurance premium surcharge
Employer B	**Smoking:** Smokers restricted to lower-value coverage option **Screening:** One site pilot program, $15 reduction in copayments
Employer C	**Screening:** $20 for completing biometric screening **HRA:** $50 for completing online health assessment **Smoking:** Up to $600 premium surcharge per year **Health goals:** $20 for achieving personal health goals
Employer D	**Screening:** Up to $2,600 annual premium differential (for individual coverage)[25] **Health outcomes:** Up to $754 annual premium differential based on biometric data and smoking status (for individual coverage)
Employer E	None offered

reported that it faced restrictions as a federal government agency, such as legal prohibitions on cash incentives for program participation, and therefore refrained from offering monetary incentives for wellness activities. It did offer an indirect incentive for improving health-related behaviors in the form of paid time off for wellness-related activities.

5.4. Types of Incentives

According to the RAND Employer Survey results, financial incentives are offered in a variety of forms, such as cash, cash equivalents (e.g., discounted gym memberships), and novelty items (e.g., t-shirts or gift cards). Novelty items were used by nearly half of all employers who offer any incentives. Gym discounts (42 percent) and cash incentives (21 percent) were cited as common way to reward program participants and/or health-related behaviors. Employers also linked cost-sharing provisions for health coverage to program participation and/or attainment of health goals, including employees' share of health plan premiums (37 percent), employer contribution to HRAs (5 percent), and cost-sharing (3 percent) (Figure 5.2).

Case studies corroborate that employers commonly offer small rewards to encourage engagement in wellness programs. All employers from our case studies reported using novelties (e.g., t-shirts, tickets to

[25] Employer D has a $50 weekly surcharge to employees' contributions to health plan premiums for employees who opt out of wellness screenings, which totals $2,600 annually.

Figure 5.2: Percentage of Employers That Use Incentives for Participation Among Employers That Have Incentives Under Their Wellness Program

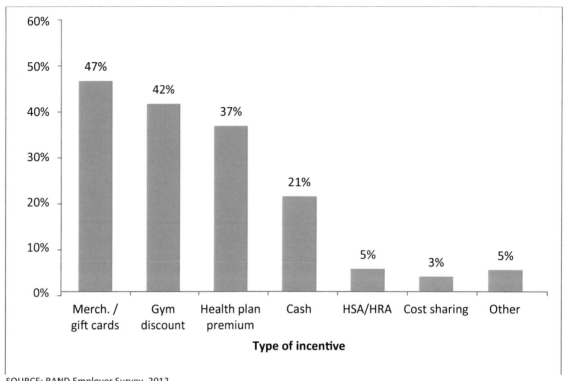

SOURCE: RAND Employer Survey, 2012.
NOTE: The graph represents information from the subset of employers with at least 50 employees that offer a wellness program (51 percent).
HSA = Health Savings Account.

events, and coffee mugs) as a strategy to engage employees. Employer A reported token incentives were used occasionally, but free massages were a popular prize. Discounted gym memberships were offered at two employer sites and administered through the health plan (Employers C and D). Employer B developed a unique approach for offering rewards; rather than targeting individual employees, raffle incentives and exercise equipment grants were sometimes offered to wellness committees to incentivize worksite wellness programs in their agencies.

Three employers in our case studies have implemented more far-reaching health plan benefit and cost-sharing structures with built-in incentives for program engagement and outcomes. For example, Employer B piloted an incentive of reduced copayments to encourage participation in a health screening. Staff received a $15 reduction in copayments for an entire year for participating in the onsite biometric screening.

As the RAND Employer Survey shows, incentives are typically framed as rewards for engaging in wellness programs. Only 2 percent of employers frame their incentive offerings only as a penalty, and 11 percent of employers reported framing incentives as penalties and rewards (Figure 5.3).

Case study findings suggest that some employers do use penalties as a way to influence health behaviors, for tobacco use in particular. Employers A and C implemented a penalty for self-reported smokers in the form of a premium surcharge, and Employer D built in higher health plan premium contributions for individuals who did not achieve specific health standards. However, it framed those penalties as "premium differentials" because of concerns that employees would view penalties negatively, and it also offered an additional premium discount for employees that met all health targets.

5.4.1. Incentive Administration

Employers can administer wellness incentives themselves, through a health plan, or both.[26] As shown in Figure 5.4, overall, approximately half of the employers handle wellness incentives themselves, about

Figure 5.3: Percentage of Incentives Framed as a Penalty, a Reward, or Both Among Employers Offering Monetary Incentives Under Their Wellness Program

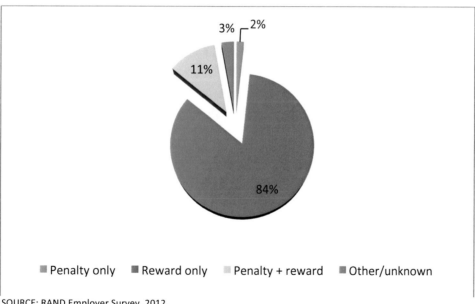

SOURCE: RAND Employer Survey, 2012.
NOTES: The graph represents information from employers with at least 50 employees that offer a monetary incentive for participation in a wellness program. 51 percent of employers offer a wellness program, and 69 percent of those have monetary incentives.

---

[26] Incentives offered by employers outside group health coverage are not subject to insurance regulations but have to comply with nondiscrimination and privacy statutes.

one-third of employers use health plans, and only about one in seven uses both methods. In addition, the RAND Employer Survey revealed that the method of incentive administration depends on the type of employee behavior that is being encouraged. Employers handle the majority of incentives for HRA completion and lifestyle management programs, whereas health plans administer the majority of incentives for disease management programs (Figure 5.4).

The method of incentive administration also varies with employment size (Figure 5.5). Small employers have the highest proportion reporting use of a health plan to manage wellness incentives. For example, the health plan administers incentives in nearly half of employers with fewer than 100 employees; in contrast, among employers with 1,000 or more employees, more than two-thirds managed wellness incentives themselves. The patterns are similar in specific programs including HRA, biometric screenings, and lifestyle management programs.

Overall, compared to other industries, companies in the trade industry tend to rely solely on health plans to administer incentives (Figure 5.6). With the exception of government agencies, approximately

Figure 5.4: Percentage Distribution of Incentive Administration for Screenings and Interventions Among Employers Offering Incentives in Their Wellness Program

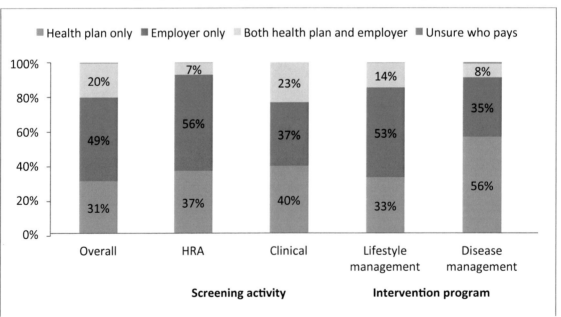

SOURCE: RAND Employer Survey, 2012.
NOTES: The graph represents information from employers with at least 50 employees that offer a monetary incentive for participation in a wellness program. 51 percent of employers offer a wellness program; of those, 65 percent have an HRA, 49 percent have clinical screenings, 77 percent have lifestyle management, and 56 percent have disease management interventions.

Figure 5.5: Percentage Distribution of Incentive Administration Among Employers Offering Incentives in Their Wellness Program, by Employer Size

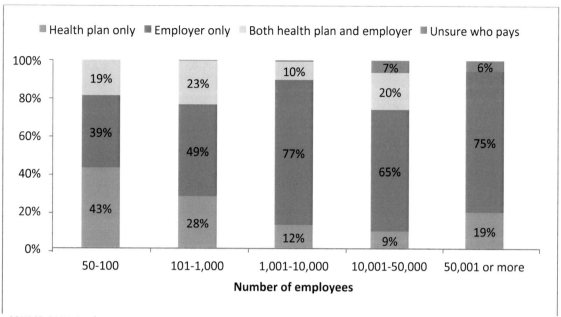

SOURCE: RAND Employer Survey, 2012.
NOTES: The graph represents information from employers with at least 50 employees that offer a monetary incentive for participation in a wellness program. 51 percent of employers offer a wellness program, and 69 percent of those have monetary incentives.

Figure 5.6: Percentage Distribution of Incentive Administration Among Employers Offering Incentives in Their Wellness Program, by Industry

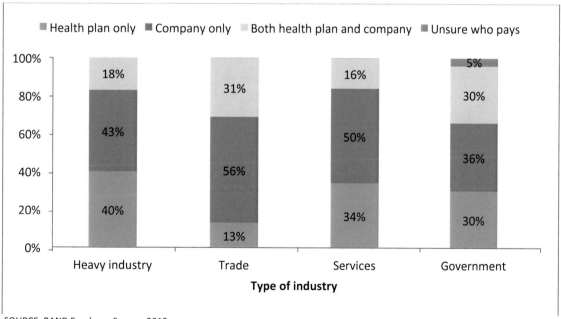

SOURCE: RAND Employer Survey, 2012.
NOTES: The graph represents information from employers with at least 50 employees that offer a monetary incentive for participation in a wellness program. 51 percent of employers offer a wellness program, and 69 percent of those have monetary incentives.

half the companies in other industries directly manage incentives. The same patterns appear in HRA and lifestyle management programs. But for biometric screenings, more than half of service industry employers use health plans only to manage incentives, but only about 15 percent to 29 percent of employers in other industries do so.

5.5. Incentives for Screening Activities

5.5.1. Prevalence and Patterns of Use

According to the RAND Employer Survey, almost half of the employers that use an HRA or biometric screening provide incentives to encourage employee participation (Figure 5.7). The median annual maximum incentive per full-time employee is $300 for participating in an HRA; however, the variation is wide, with approximately one-third of employers (31 percent) offering less than $100 and only 15 percent offering more than $1,000, as seen in Figure 5.8. Similar incentive amounts are offered for participation in clinical screening (Figure 5.9).

According to data for five employers in the CCA database, incentive amounts for HRA completion ranged from $50 to $100, as listed in Table 5.2. Of note, Employer 2 started using incentives in 2009 but

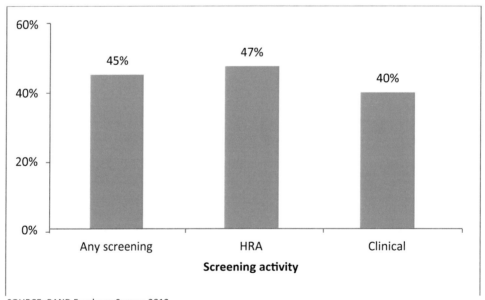

Figure 5.7: Percentage of Employers That Offer Incentives for Screenings Among Employers Providing Any Screening Activities

SOURCE: RAND Employer Survey, 2012.
NOTES: The graph represents information from employers with at least 50 employees that offer a monetary incentive for participation in a screening activity component of a wellness program. 51 percent of employers offer a wellness program; of those, 80 percent have screening activities, 65 percent have an HRA, and 49 percent have clinical screenings.

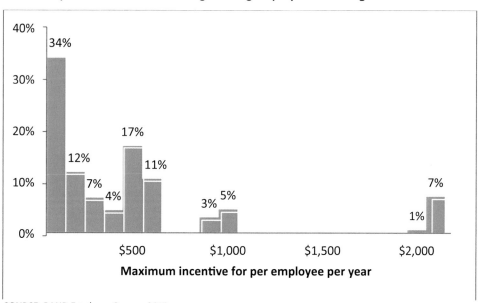

Figure 5.8: Percentage Distribution of Maximum Annual Incentive Amounts for HRA Completion Among Employers Providing Such Incentives

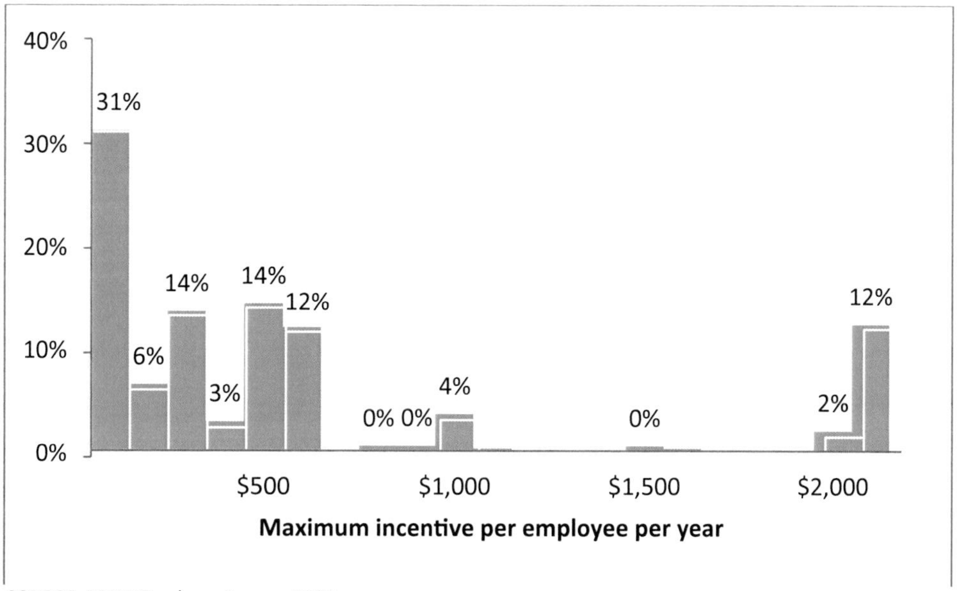

SOURCE: RAND Employer Survey, 2012.
NOTES: The graph represents information from employers with at least 50 employees that offer a monetary incentive for participation in an HRA as a component of a wellness program. 51 percent of employers offer a wellness program, 65 percent of those have an HRA, and 47 percent of those offer a monetary incentive. Incentive amounts greater than $2,000 were combined for visibility.

Figure 5.9: Percentage Distribution of Maximum Annual Incentive Amounts for Participation in Clinical Screenings Among Employers Providing Such Incentives

SOURCE: RAND Employer Survey, 2012.
NOTES: The graph represents information from employers with at least 50 employees that offer a monetary incentive for participation in clinical screening as a component of a wellness program. 51 percent of employers offer a wellness program, 49 percent of those have clinical screenings, and 40 percent of those offer a monetary incentive. Incentive amounts greater than $2,000 were combined to enhance visibility.

Table 5.2: Incentives Offered by Employers 1–5 for HRA Completion, by Year

Employer	Incentive Amount ($)				
	2006	2007	2008	2009	2010
1	0	0	75	75	75
2	0	0	0	50	0
3	0	0	0	100	100
4	0	50	50	50	–
5	0	100	100	100	100

SOURCE: RAND analysis of health plan claims and screening and wellness program data in the CCA database.
NOTE: "–" denotes that data on incentives are not available for that year.

discontinued them in 2010. Four employers paid out incentives in cash, and Employer 5 used an insurance premium deduction.

5.5.2. Impact on Wellness Screening Participation

A simulation model shows that the incentive amount for HRA completion had a significant effect on completion rates. On average, an increase in the HRA incentive by $10 is associated with a 1.6 percentage point increase in the HRA completion rate. As shown in Figure 5.10, our results suggest that a completion rate of about 40 percent would be expected for an employer without any incentive for HRA completion, whereas a 57 percent completion rate would be expected with an incentive of $100.

Figure 5.10: Percentage Distribution of Simulated Effect of Incentive Amounts on HRA Completion Rates in the CCA Analytic Sample

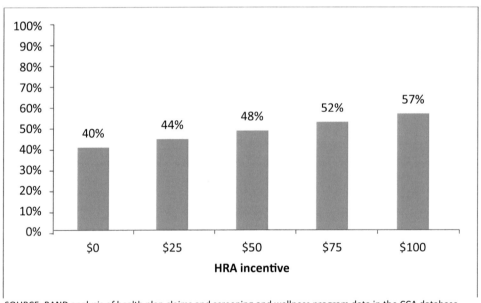

SOURCE: RAND analysis of health plan claims and screening and wellness program data in the CCA database.
NOTE: Analysis of CCA data for Employers 1–5; $p < 0.01$.

Although no employers in our case studies conducted formal evaluations of the impact of incentives on employee participation in screening activities, feedback from two employer sites indicates that employees are motivated by monetary incentives. Employer D first rolled out voluntary onsite preventive screenings but found that participation rates were lower than anticipated, hovering around 20 percent and attracting only the most health conscious employees, in the opinion of our interviewees. In 2009, the company implemented a weekly $50 insurance premium surcharge for employees who did not participate in screenings. The new incentive program resulted in nearly 100 percent participation. A focus group participant reported, "[We] all do it [complete screenings] because [we] don't want to have to pay that extra $50" and "it's expensive!"

Focus group participants at Employer C reported that the small monetary incentive influences their decision to participate in onsite screenings, "You walk in there, you get $20. I mean, it's free money." Organizational leaders also stated that modest incentives were successful at "catching employees' attentions" but that raising the amount would not have much effect.

5.6. Incentives for Interventions

5.6.1. Prevalence and Patterns of Use

Employers use incentives to encourage participation in lifestyle management programs almost as much as in HRA completion. The RAND Employer Survey data suggest that almost 40 percent of employers with a lifestyle management program offer financial incentives to encourage participation (Figure 5.11). However, employers use incentives for disease management program participation much less frequently (7 percent).

Incentives for lifestyle management programs are offered more often and with a larger incentive amount than for disease management programs. Two-thirds (71 percent) of employers offer their eligible employees an opportunity to receive more than $200 for participation in lifestyle management programs. Figure 5.12 provides the breakdown by amount. This is more than twice the proportion of employers offering $200 or more for participation in disease management (Figure 5.13).

Within lifestyle management programs, incentives for smoking, weight management, and fitness are most commonly offered (Figure 5.14). According to the RAND Employer Survey data, about a quarter of

Figure 5.11: Percentage of Employers with a Wellness Program That Offer Incentives for Participation in Interventions

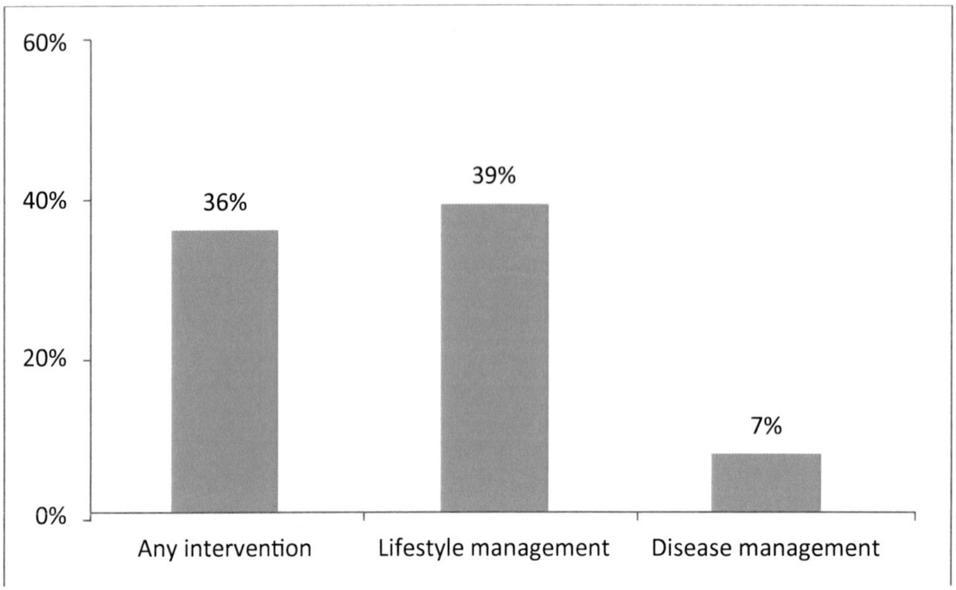

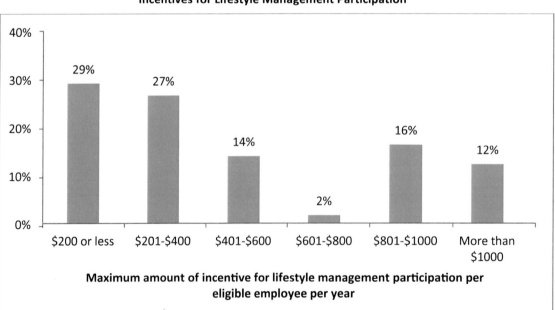

SOURCE: RAND Employer Survey, 2012.
NOTES: The graph represents information from employers with at least 50 employees that offer a monetary incentive for participation in an intervention component of a wellness program. 51 percent of employers offer a wellness program; of those, 80 percent have interventions, 77 percent have lifestyle management interventions, and 56 percent have disease management interventions.

Figure 5.12: Percentage Distribution of Maximum Annual Incentive Amounts Offered for Participation in Lifestyle Management Programs Among Employers Providing Any Incentives for Lifestyle Management Participation

SOURCE: RAND Employer Survey, 2012.
NOTES: The graph represents information from employers with at least 50 employees that offer a monetary incentive for participation in any lifestyle management intervention as a component of a wellness program. 51 percent of those employers offer a wellness program, 77 percent of those have any lifestyle management intervention, and 30 percent of those offer a financial incentive.

Figure 5.13: Percentage Distribution of Maximum Annual Incentive Amounts Offered for Participation in Disease Management Programs Among Employers Providing Any Incentives for Disease Management

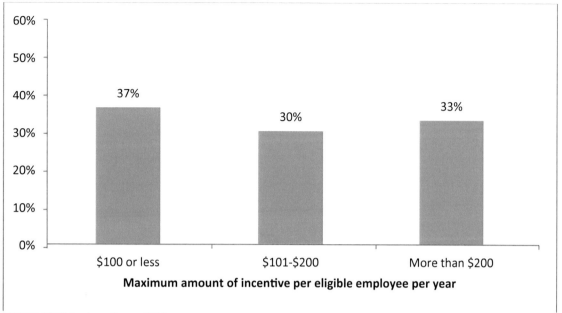

SOURCE: RAND Employer Survey, 2012.
NOTES: The graph represents information from employers with at least 50 employees that offer a monetary incentive for participation in any disease management intervention as a component of a wellness program. 51 percent of employers offer a wellness program, 56 percent of those have any lifestyle management intervention, and 4 percent of those offer a financial incentive.

Figure 5.14: Percentage of Employers That Use Incentives to Target Behaviors Among Employers Offering Incentives for Lifestyle Management Interventions in Their Wellness Program

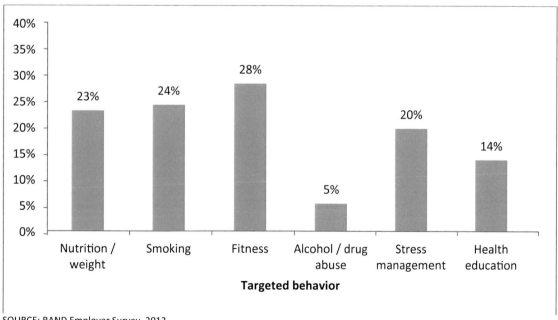

SOURCE: RAND Employer Survey, 2012.
NOTES: The graph represents information from employers with at least 50 employees that offer a monetary incentive for participation in lifestyle management for the targeted behavior as a component of a wellness program. 51 percent of employers offer a wellness program, and 77 percent of those have lifestyle management. Among employers with a lifestyle management intervention, 79 percent target nutrition/weight, 77 percent target smoking, 72 percent have fitness programs, 52 percent target alcohol/drug abuse, 52 percent have stress management programs, and 36 percent offer health education.

employers who target those risks/behaviors offer incentives to promote program participation. Participation rates are consistently higher among employers who use monetary incentives in lifestyle management. For smoking cessation programs, the participation rate for programs with incentives (10 percent) is twice that of programs without incentives (5 percent). For fitness programs, the participation rate is approximately one-half greater (26 percent compared to 18 percent).

Although four of the five employers in our case studies used some type of financial incentives to promote wellness program participation and behavior change, wellness program managers had mixed feelings about use of incentives to encourage healthy behaviors. Some expert interviewees reported that employees were motivated by health insurance premium surcharges for smokers knowing that they "could save a few dollars through good behavior" and treating it as a "tipping point" to quit smoking. At the same time, at Employer A, we learned that program staff members do not believe that participation in wellness activities should be incentivized financially; rather, the strongest motivator should be the desire to be healthy and fit. As a wellness program representative put it, "when it comes to changing your health, the real motivation has to be internal, and you have to want it. To help them, we need to build their awareness, and that's what we're trying to promote here. If somebody forced me to participate, or if people participated to get an iPod or something like that, I don't know how genuine that participation is. I think that's a struggle in the wellness field in general." As described in this quote, the wellness program's goal is to build awareness about healthy lifestyles and to provide resources necessary to help employees stay healthy and fit.

According to the RAND Employer Survey results, employers with smoking cessation programs are almost as likely to reward program participation (24 percent) as actual smoking cessation (19 percent). In contrast, incentives for weight management and fitness programs are much more likely to be tied to attaining health goals. About a quarter of employers reported using incentives for participation in weight control and fitness programs, whereas only 3 and 6 percent, respectively, used incentives for reaching targets (or an alternative standard) (Figure 5.15). Results-based incentives are more commonly administered by the employer directly than through the health plan.

Case study findings are consistent with survey results in that they show that participation-based incentives are more common than outcome-based incentives. For example, four of five case study

Figure 5.15: Percentage of Employers with Wellness Programs Using Participation and Results-Based Incentives for Selected Health Behaviors

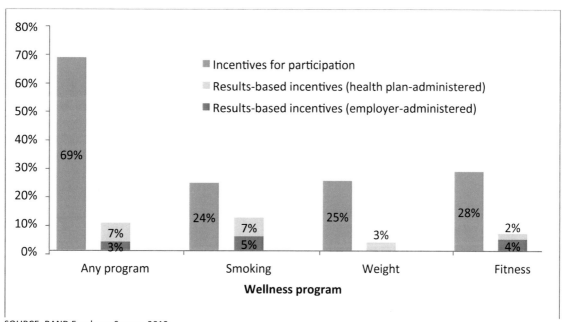

SOURCE: RAND Employer Survey, 2012.

NOTES: The graph represents information from employers with at least 50 employees that offer monetary incentives for participation in lifestyle management interventions. 51 percent of employers offer a wellness program, and 77 percent of those have lifestyle management. Among employers with a lifestyle management intervention, 77 percent target smoking, 79 percent target weight management, and 72 percent offer fitness programs.

employers (A, B, C, and D) impose smoking penalties on their employees, in the form of higher health insurance premiums, if they do not attempt to quit smoking, whereas only Employers D and E used any incentives under their wellness programs for behaviors or health targets other than smoking. It is worth noting that Employer E uses only indirect rewards for increasing healthy behaviors in the form of paid time off for fitness and other wellness-related activities, such as attending health education classes. Finally, only Employer D ties premium costs to an employee's ability to meet specific health outcomes, such as blood pressure, tobacco/nicotine use, cholesterol, or BMI, which are assessed annually during onsite screenings.

Smoking is the only health risk for which achieving the goal is rewarded with a higher incentive than participation in a program. The average incentive ($682) paid out for stopping tobacco use is more than triple the incentive paid out for program participation ($203) (Figure 5.16).

Using data from the RAND Employer Survey, we estimate that approximately 7 percent of employers that offer wellness programs administer results-based incentives through their health plans.

Figure 5.16: Average Annual Incentive Amounts Paid by Employers Offering Incentives

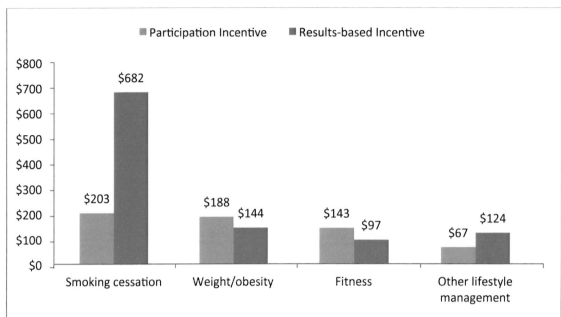

SOURCE: RAND Employer Survey, 2012.
NOTES: The graph represents information from employers with at least 50 employees that offer monetary incentives for participation in lifestyle management interventions. 51 percent of employers offer a wellness program, and 77 percent of those have lifestyle management. Among employers with a lifestyle management intervention, 77 percent target smoking, 79 percent target weight management, and 72 percent offer fitness programs.

When looking at the individual survey responses of the 12 employers, who provided information on the maximum results-based incentives offered to employees and the average monthly cost of their health plan premiums, we find that the maximum incentives offered by those 12 employers range from $120 to ten times that amount (Figure 5.17). The average maximum incentive amount for these employers was less than 10 percent of the total annual cost of coverage, far from the current 20 percent regulatory threshold. None of the employers in our survey reported incentive amounts exceeding this threshold (Figure 5.18).

These findings are supported by our case study results. Two case study employers impose a $50 monthly insurance premium surcharge on those employees who self-identify themselves as smokers and report that they do not intend to quit smoking (Employer C), or do not participate in a free smoking cessation program, or do not use free smoking cessation products (Employer A). Moreover, employees of Employer D (the only employer that uses outcome-based incentives) who complete the annual biometric health screening but do not achieve the required standards have a premium surcharge of $6.25 or $12.50 per week, depending on the number of goals they do not meet. Employees who meet all goals receive a $2 credit each week. Therefore the maximum surcharge is $14.50 per week or $754

Figure 5.17: Maximum Annual Incentive Amounts Offered by Health Plans for Achieving Health Goals

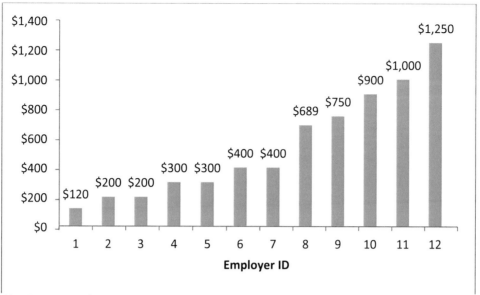

SOURCE: RAND Employer Survey, 2012.
NOTE: The graph represents nonweighted results based on information from employers that reported incentive amounts offered by health plans for employees that achieve health goals.

Figure 5.18: Percentage of the Maximum Annual Incentive Amount Offered by Health Plans for Achieving Health Goals Relative to the Annual Cost of Coverage, by Employer ID

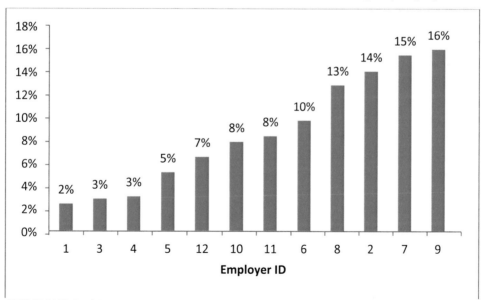

SOURCE: RAND Employer Survey, 2012.
NOTES: The graph represents nonweighted results based on information from employers that reported monthly premiums and incentive amounts offered by health plans for employees that achieve health goals. Percentage of annual premium = (annual maximum incentive amount per employee/annual monthly premium per employee) * 12 months.

per year.[27] Employees can obtain a waiver from their physician, if it is not medically advisable for them to meet the targets. Wellness program managers at Employer D purposely intended to stay away from the 20 percent regulatory threshold. Furthermore, they are in the process of putting less emphasis on health standards by implementing financial incentives for reaching incremental health goals, such as losing five pounds, rather than achieving specific results, such as a target BMI.

5.6.2. Impact of Incentives on Program Participation

Four employers in the CCA database had sufficient information with which to evaluate the use of incentives on wellness program participation, but none of them reported using incentives tied to actual behavior change or health goal attainment. The annual incentive amounts ranged from $50 to $125 and are listed in Table 5.3. All incentives were paid as cash. Of note, Employer 2 discontinued the use of incentives in 2010.

Because of the limited variation in incentive use, our multivariate analyses on the effect of incentives on lifestyle program participation did not generate stable results. We therefore do not present them here.

Employer C in our case studies offered a $50 monetary incentive for participation in lifestyle management programs administered through the health plan; however, reported participation rates

Table 5.3: Incentives Offered by Employers 1–4 for Program Participation

Employer	Incentive Amount ($)				
	2006	2007	2008	2009	2010
1	0	0	125	125	75
2	0	0	0	50	0
3	0	0	0	0	100
4	0	0	0	0	–

SOURCE: RAND analysis of health plan claims and screening and wellness program data in the CCA database.
NOTE: "–" denotes that data on incentives were not available.

[27] HIPAA permits employers to offer incentives based on outcomes of up to 20 percent of the total annual cost of coverage. The cost of coverage (for a single individual) at Employer D is estimated at $7,096; therefore, the maximum results-based surcharge of $14.50 per week, or $754 per year, is approximately 11 percent of the cost of coverage.

were low and the impact of these incentives were not assessed. Focus group participants stated that these small monetary incentives did not motivate them to engage in programs, and changes in their health behavior were driven by intrinsic motivation rather than rewards.

5.6.3. Impact of Incentives on Health-Related Behaviors and Outcomes

Regression results suggest that incentives are associated with improvements in smoking, BMI, and exercise but not in cholesterol levels. Although the relationship between incentive levels and the three behaviors/outcomes is statistically significant, the magnitude of the effect is small. We estimate that, in the range of incentives observed in our data set ($0 to $200), for every $10 in incentives, BMI decreases by 0.004 kg/m2, which corresponds to a weight loss of 0.03 pounds for the average adult male (Figure 5.19). Similarly, $10 in additional incentives is associated with 0.01 additional days with more than 20 minutes of exercise and a 0.4 percentage point reduction in the smoking rate.

Our analyses were hindered by the small number of employers available for analysis (Employers 1–5 depending on analysis), as well as limited variation in incentives across employers and over time.

In two employers in our case studies, incentives were tied to health outcomes. Employer C offers $20 for employees who achieve an individualized health goal (e.g., lose five pounds in six weeks or exercise

Figure 5.19: Simulated impact of Incentive Amounts on BMI in the CCA Analytic Sample

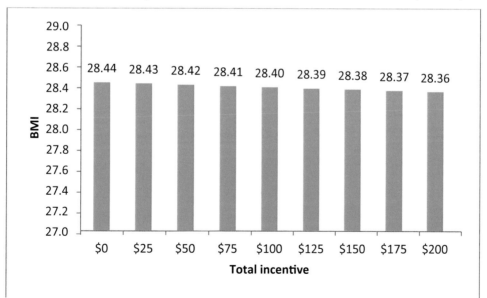

SOURCE: RAND analysis of health plan claims and screening and wellness program data in the CCA database.
NOTE: Analysis of CCA data for Employers 1 and 3; p < 0.01.

three times weekly for two months), which is set based on employee health assessment and other personal needs. The organization did not conduct a formal assessment of the impact of these incentives on motivating behavior change and improving health, but focus group participants shared that the small rewards had only a limited impact on their behavior and that stronger incentives would not influence their decisions any more.

Moreover, focus group participants at Employer D did not report employee premium differentials as a motivator to change their health behavior; in fact, many regarded the premium differential as given and were unaware of the link between screening results and employee premium contributions. In contrast, executives, who were well informed about the program, reported that they were motivated by the premium surcharge, knowing that they "could save a few dollars through good behavior." Another organizational leader admitted that the premium surcharge was a "tipping point" to help him quit smoking.

5.7. Discussion of the Current Use of Incentives

5.7.1. Overall Uptake

Over two-thirds of employers in the RAND Employer Survey reported using incentives to promote employee engagement in worksite wellness programs. The frequent use is confirmed by the KFF/HRET (2012) survey reporting that 41 percent of employers with more than 200 employees used such incentives in 2012 (KFF/HRET, 2012). This practice is not confined to the private sector; a recent review suggested that states are beginning to offer incentives for participation or goal attainment for their workers (Hoffman, 2012).

Incentive use also appears to be increasing over time and therefore would be expected to continue to increase in the near future. Mercer Consulting's National Survey of Employer-Sponsored Health Plans estimated that in 2009, 21 percent of employers with 500 or more employees provided financial incentives for participating in at least one wellness program (Mercer, 2010), and that the number had risen to 33 percent by 2011 (Mercer, 2011). Similarly, data from the KFF/HRET (2010) survey indicate that 23 percent of employers offered any incentives for wellness program engagement in 2010 (KFF/HRET, 2010) and 41 percent in 2012 (KFF/HRET, 2012). In the RAND Employer Survey, a total of 33 percent of employers not offering incentives planned to do so, and 20 percent of employers already offering incentives want to increase the amounts. The 2012 Mercer survey confirms this finding, suggesting that as many as 87 percent of employers with more than 200 employees plan to add or strengthen incentive programs (Mercer, 2011).

It is also expected that the magnitude of incentives will increase. In the RAND Employer Survey, about a quarter of employers currently using incentives plan to offer additional incentives for participation, completion, and health results. In addition, 15 percent indicated interest in increasing the amount of incentives for program participation. A 2011 nonrepresentative membership survey of the National Business Group on Health, a coalition of large employers, found that 19 percent of employers intend to increase the maximum incentive amount in 2014, when the new regulations come into effect (Darling, Dannel and Lykens, 2011).

5.7.2. Role of Incentives for Screening Activities

Data from the RAND Employer Survey reveal that employers use incentives commonly to increase employee participation in wellness screening activities, such as health risk assessments. Similarly, the KFF/HRET survey data found that in 2010, 36 percent of employers with more than 200 employees, who offered an HRA, provided a financial incentive for completion and that the number had increased to 63 percent by 2012. (KFF/HRET, 2010; KFF/HRET, 2012) This emphasis on HRA completion reflects the critical role of data both to identify individual health risks and to direct employees to appropriate resources and to help employers plan and evaluate wellness programs. At the same time, completing a short questionnaire imposes little burden on employees, and our case study feedback suggests that employees accept the need to provide the information. The analysis of the CCA data indicates that incentives for HRA completion are effective, particularly above a threshold of $50.

5.7.3. Role of Incentives for Program Participation

According to the RAND Employer Survey, incentives are commonly used for participation in lifestyle management inventions, particularly for interventions that target smoking, diet, and exercise, whereas incentives are used infrequently for disease management interventions. Because of the limited information on program eligibility in the CCA database, we were unable to estimate the impact of incentives on participation rates. However, the RAND Employer Survey data suggest that rates of participation in intervention programs are higher for employers that use program incentives.

5.7.4. Role of Incentives for Achieving Health Standards

The proper use of incentives to further health goal attainment is currently subject to a lively debate among policymakers, researchers, legal experts, employers, and employees. The debate is centered on whether such incentives are legally permissible, whether they are effective, whether they are ethical, and whether they can have unintended consequences (Madison, Volpp and Halpern, 2011). On the first question, a recent review found that the Affordable Care Act has clarified the range of legally permissible incentives at the federal level and that state laws are beginning to mirror federal standards (Klautzer, Mattke and Greenberg, 2012). There is much less clarity on the other questions, given that incentives for health outcomes are a recent phenomenon, their use remains limited, especially large monetary incentives, and the empirical literature scant (Volpp et al., 2011).

Data from the RAND Employer Survey conducted as part of this study provides national estimates for the use of results-based incentives among employers with 50 or more employees. The data indicate that incentives tied to health standards primarily target smoking cessation. Employers with smoking cessation programs are almost as likely to reward program participation (21 percent) as actual smoking cessation (19 percent), whereas employers were three to four times more likely to reward participation in other health risk intervention programs (e.g., weight management program) than behavior change or outcomes (e.g., weight loss). Similarly, four out of five case study employers penalized smokers, but only two had incentives for other health standards, and for one of the two, the incentive was only $20 to reach a self-selected target. Smoking is also the only health risk for which actual behavior change is tied to higher monetary incentives than those for program participation, according to both survey data and our case studies.

According to the scientific literature, there is mixed evidence on the impact of financial incentives on motivating smoking cessation (Cahill and Perera, 2011; Osilla et al., 2012), and a 2011 review of the literature concluded that financial incentives may attract individuals to enroll or participate in programs but do not achieve long-term behavior change (Cahill and Perera, 2011). One randomized control trial found that large incentives (of up to $750 over the course of a year) were effective in improving abstinence rates. In particular, this review found that a $400 cash reward for sustained abstinence at 12 months resulted in increased abstinence (Volpp et al., 2009).

A growing literature supports designing incentive schemes that reward participants for making progress toward health goals rather than meeting stringent health standards (Schmidt, 2012). One case study employer developed an incentive scheme based on achieving specific health standards, such as achieving a target BMI, but has since modified its strategy to reward employees for making improvements in their health, such as losing five pounds. This type of incentive design may encourage individuals to improve their health status rather than achieve goals that might otherwise seem unattainable (Schmidt, 2012).

We also find that results-based incentives are more commonly administered by the employer directly rather than through the health plan and linked to coverage. According to the RAND Employer Survey, about 7 percent of employers that offer wellness programs reported administering results-based incentives through their health plans. The average amount of results-based incentives for these employers was less than 10 percent of the total cost of health coverage, far from the current regulatory threshold.

With respect to effectiveness, our analyses of employer data in the CCA database show that incentives for HRA completion and program participation can significantly reduce weight and smoking rates and increase exercise. However, the size of these effects is small and unlikely to be clinically meaningful. None of the employers in our case studies had formally evaluated the effect of their results-based incentives.

5.7.5. Limitations

As we pointed out in the previous section, the employers in the CCA database and our case studies are not necessarily representative of all employers, which limits the generalizability of our results. Further, the limited variation in incentive levels among employers in the CCA database restricts our ability to detect any meaningful effects, and we cannot extrapolate effects beyond the maximum level of $200 that was observed in the data. The limited variation in incentive levels also made it impossible to test statistically whether different incentive types (e.g., cash rewards or premium discounts) have a differential effect. Although we are confident that the analytic methods are appropriate, residual bias in our estimates cannot be ruled out, given the nonexperimental nature of our research.

5.7.6. Conclusion

Financial incentives have become a commonly used tool to promote employee engagement in worksite wellness programs, and employers are expanding their use. To date the most common trigger for incentives is participation in screening activities, and our results suggest that such incentives, particularly above $50, are effective. Incentives are also commonly used to increase participation in wellness interventions, such as weight loss programs, but the evidence for their effectiveness remains weak. A smaller number of employers tie incentives to achieving health standards, which primarily target smoking cessation. We find a statistically significant but small effect of incentives up to $200 on weight loss, exercise, and smoking, but potential unintended consequences of such incentives, in particular on vulnerable employees, cannot be ruled out given current evidence. More research on how to craft incentives to achieve desired program goals is needed.

Chapter 6: Lessons from Case Studies for Program Implementation

To better understand how workplace wellness programs are implemented in practice and how participating employees view such programs, we identified common themes across the five case study employers and the literature. This chapter describes approaches employers used for implementing program interventions and key factors that promote wellness program success.

6.1. Program Modalities

Interventions under workplace wellness programs can be categorized into two groups, individual-level interventions, which target the specific health risks of individual workers, and public health strategies, which target the entire workforce collectively. Typically, employers use both types of interventions to achieve program goals.

6.1.1. Individual-Level Interventions

For interventions at the individual level, employers typically collect data about the health risk factors of individual employees through an HRA or biometric screening and link employees to appropriate interventions based on the results of the screening (Figure 6.1). In three of five employers (C, D, and E) from our case studies, workers are linked to interventions through "gateways," such as HRAs or

Figure 6.1: Typical Employer Activities Related to Employee Health Interventions

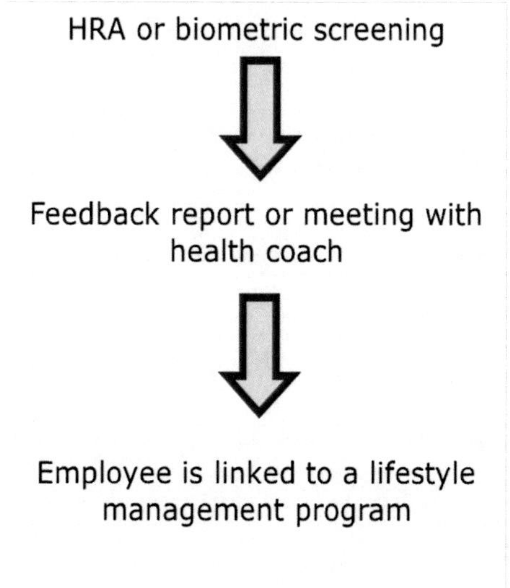

HRA or biometric screening

Feedback report or meeting with health coach

Employee is linked to a lifestyle management program

biometric screenings. The interventions are then provided to individual employees or groups of employees. Examples of interventions are nutritional counseling or smoking cessation counseling, both of which were offered at all five case study employers.

6.1.2. Interventions for the Entire Workforce

Workforce-level interventions target all members in the organization's workforce, rather than individual employees. They aim to promote healthy behaviors and develop a culture of wellness for the entire workforce. Examples include educational campaigns, such as "lunch-and-learn" sessions on nutrition, subsidizing entry fees into running events, and holding organization-wide health fairs. Commonly, public health approaches include modifications in the workplace to encourage healthy behaviors—for instance, offering healthier snack options in the vending machines or hanging signs by the elevator to encourage employees to take the stairs.

All five employers in the case studies introduced some workforce interventions within their organization. For example, Employer B's wellness program coordinated with a local farmer to sell fresh local produce to employees once a week and offers a low-cost healthy lunch special. Three employers made healthier meals and snacks more available. Four employers (A, B, C, and D) have begun offering healthier food choices in vending machines or the cafeteria.

6.2. Key Factors for Workplace Wellness Programs

Through our case studies and literature review, we identified five common factors that can promote wellness program success. Although the actual impact of these factors has yet to be evaluated empirically, five common themes emerged from our review.

6.2.1. Develop Effective Communication Strategies

All five organizations in our case studies employ strategies to communicate wellness program information to employees, ranging from face-to-face interaction to mass dissemination to ensure that employees know which programs and services are available to them and that they understand how to access them.

Table 6.1: Five Key Factors That Promote Wellness Program Success

Factors	Description
Effective communication strategies	Outreach strategy entails use of multiple communication channels to ensure that employees know the services that are available and how to access them; organizational leaders deliver clear messages about the importance and goals of programs.
Opportunity for employees to engage	Activities are convenient, easily accessible, and address the underlying needs of targeted employees.
Leadership engaged at all levels	Senior management views wellness as an organizational priority and invests in building a culture of wellness; direct supervisors respond to the needs of workers, generate excitement, and connect employees to available resources.
Use of existing resources and relationships	Organization leverages existing resources and builds relationships, often with health plans to expand offerings at little to no cost.
Continuous evaluation	Organization conducts employee needs assessments, continually improves feedback processes, and evaluates program outcomes.

6.2.1.a. Broad Communication Outreach

Employers cited the importance of using multiple communication channels, especially for those organizations with a large, and geographically dispersed, workforce. All employers used posters or bulletin boards in the workplace to deliver information about programs or reminders about the importance of healthy behaviors. All five organizations create awareness through health and wellness–themed newsletters, and four employers have held such events as health fairs to raise the profile of their wellness activities.

A program manager at Employer B noted that, although very cost-effective and convenient, email is not the only way to advertise activities: "supervisors may have email, but floor workers don't and that's a big working class at [the facility]." Wellness program staff members thus ask supervisors to post flyers, make announcements during staff meetings, and put information on bulletin boards. For larger announcements, the director of the workplace facility often sends out email to supervisors to promote the event.

The program at Employer D, a manufacturing firm, uses a similar multichannel communication strategy to reach its diversified workforce. Flyers to announce upcoming competitions and notices of annual onsite screenings are posted in break rooms at the plants and dropped in employees' mailboxes. The wellness portal on the company's Intranet, which is "consistently updated with wellness news and events," was a primary way to communicate to employees in the corporate office with easy access to email. However, both manufacturing and corporate workers admitted that they often overlook email communications or did not recall seeing flyers or other communication materials regarding wellness.

In contrast, a wellness website is the most comprehensive source for describing wellness programs at Employer E. Activities are listed on the website's calendar, and employees can opt to receive targeted emails announcing upcoming classes that may pertain to them based on their HRA results. However, because many manufacturing employees have limited computer access while at work, they tend to be less aware of program offerings than are the white collar office workers.

Employer C illustrates how lack of communication can negatively impact uptake:

> The organization promotes the onsite biometric screening through signage, newsletters and email reminders, and offers a small monetary incentive for completion ($20). Employees in our focus group indicated a high level of awareness of the screening events, and executives confirmed high participation rates. Conversely, the employer's health plan offered a $50 incentive for completion of an online HRA, but the availability of this program component was not widely advertised. As a result, many focus group participants stated that they were unaware of the HRA and had never completed it, even though the incentive amount was higher than that offered for undergoing biometric screening.

A catchy name helps a program to be successful. According to a wellness program representative at Employer A, using catchy program titles draws people's attention and helps them remember about wellness activities offered in the workplace: "People do seem to gravitate to programs, if they can remember their names."

6.2.1.b. Clear Communication About Goals of Wellness Interventions

Program success requires that organizational leaders deliver clear messages about the importance and goals of the wellness programs. One case study employer (D) provides an example of how a multifaceted program with both an onsite screening and lifestyle interventions fell short of its mission to educate employees about their health status and instead resulted in a misunderstanding among employees about the purpose of the wellness program:

> The organization rolled-out annual onsite biometric screening in conjunction with a number of friendly weight-loss and nutritional competitions with the intent to not only

educate employees of their health risks, but encourage them to participate in activities to foster healthy behavior change. A third party vendor was responsible for communicating messages about onsite screenings, while messages on wellness activities came from internal sources, such as direct supervisors, executives and employee champions.

These various communication channels appear to have unintentionally created confusion among employees. The employer intended the onsite screening paired with premium adjustments as a tool to inform individuals of their health status; however, focus group participants did not recognize wellness screenings as a component of the wellness program. When queried about screenings, one focus group participant responded, "That's not the wellness program, that's our insurance." Another employee commented, "The screening, yeah, we have to do it for insurance." Employees perceived such wellness activities as weight-loss competitions and nutritional tracking as the "wellness program," while considering the screenings as a necessity to obtain health coverage, rather than as a way to create awareness for health risks. According to feedback from focus group participants, the screenings tied to premium adjustments may fall short of their mission to raise awareness and spur behavior change as organizational leaders had intended.

6.2.2. Ensure That All Employees Have an Opportunity to Engage

Even well-developed programs will not achieve optimal results without the active engagement of employees. Employees are more inclined to participate in wellness activities if they are convenient and address the underlying needs of targeted employees.

6.2.2.a. Program Accessibility

Those included in the case study discussions revealed that making wellness activities convenient and easily accessible for all employees are strategies that employers use to raise the level of employee engagement. Employer A offers individualized health coaching that participants can schedule in their own offices or at nearby locations as well as massage services and meditation classes, which are offered in a variety of locations. One focus group participant at a large service organization (Employer C) shared that access to the workout facility allows him to incorporate exercise into his daily routine and provides an outlet for stress relief: "I do go down to the gym and I found that that's a break that I could use, but I also found that just the convenience of it helped me."

98

In contrast, some focus group participants have limited access to wellness benefits because of their work schedules or wait times. Employer E, a large government organization that employs both blue collar and office workers, implemented a fitness benefit that allows employees to exercise or attend health-related classes three hours per week during their work day. White collar employees, who enjoy greater flexibility of hours and schedules, took advantage of the fitness benefit, whereas access for maintenance workers was commonly limited by work schedules and mandatory overtime. Most wellness classes and services were offered during the day shift, reducing access for other employees.

A manufacturing firm (Employer D) promotes healthy eating by providing discounts at Subway during the lunch hour; however, manufacturing employees are hourly workers and do not have sufficient break time to take advantage of this benefit. "[I] couldn't get to Subway and back [in time] . . . because it's all the way across town." Focus group participants at both employers reported that this unequal access contributes to tensions in the workforce and dissatisfaction.

Employees at a large service organization (Employer C) with flexible work schedules cited long wait times as a deterrent to their participation in onsite screenings. One employee complained that onsite biometric screenings can be "a nuisance" because of unpredictable wait times, which has discouraged participation: "If there's a long line—it's not worth waiting for."

Additionally, reasonable accommodations for persons with disabilities (e.g., offering classes at accessible, ADA-compliant sites and providing informational material in plain language and alternate formats, such as large print) are important to ensure accessibility; however case study employers did not discuss tailoring wellness programs to the needs of people with disabilities.

6.2.2.b. Alignment of Wellness Activities with Employee Preferences

Effective wellness programs require that managers implement programs that address the preferences of employees. Interviews with employees and executives at a manufacturing firm (Employer D) indicated, for example, that leaders' perceptions of effective wellness interventions are misaligned with employees' needs, which created divisiveness among employees:

> Executives in the corporate office revealed a strong interest in implementing wellness activities to encourage physical activity, while employees reported exercise as a lesser

priority to improve their health because they "work twelve hours . . . and have been on their feet all day." Focus group participants expressed a strong desire to have increased access to healthy food at the worksite. One focus group participant suggested heavier foods be replaced by "bananas and angel food cake" during workplace parties and fruit be available rather than snack food in break rooms.

Conversely, focus group participants at Employer A felt that program offerings were wide-ranging and met the needs of most individuals in the diverse workforce. As one employee put it, "almost anything that I could possibly want is either available or they would have available." The program is constantly adding new components and leaders are looking for innovative approaches to promote healthy activities among staff.

6.2.3. Engage Leadership to Cultivate a Culture of Wellness That Thrives

We learned that a strong commitment at all levels of the organization is important to ensure program visibility and employee buy-in. All five employers in our case study agreed that leaders must view wellness as an organizational priority and invest in building a culture of wellness to achieve optimal results.

6.2.3.a. Strong Support of Senior Managers

Evidence from our case studies suggests that employers consider support from leaders a crucial component of program development and operations. Employer C reported that senior managers understand the business case for workplace wellness program and consider it a strategic priority. One human resource representative reported, "We have full support of leadership," which has been helpful for wellness leaders as they have developed their programs. "[Managers] understand why this makes sense from a business perspective; [this] has helped create a culture of health." Focus group participants agreed that senior leaders "practice what they preach" by taking the initiative to improve their own health and fitness, which cultivates a supportive work culture.

Similarly, Employer D articulated wellness as a corporate responsibility and had the desire to "improve wellness culture" and "promote awareness" of health that can be measured only in "soft dollars." One leader shared that as health care costs are rising, implementing wellness was necessary to ensure the financial sustainability not only of the company but also the community at large: "I grew up in this community, it's important to me to have jobs available within our community and for [the company] to continue to be viable as a business in general so we can continue to employ individuals."

100

To supplement support from leadership, Employer D identifies employees as "wellness champions" to generate enthusiasm about wellness activities and communicate health-related messages, particularly to "employees in the production field [i.e., away from the main worksites] who are difficult to reach."

6.2.3.b. Wholehearted Buy-In of Direct Supervisors

Evidence from our case studies indicates that organizational leaders rely on direct supervisors to respond to the needs of workers, generate excitement for programs, and connect employees to available resources. However, four of five employers (A, C, D, and E) indicated that mid-level managers are sometimes viewed as unenthusiastic supporters or are unengaged in wellness programs. At a large university (Employer A), there was consensus among focus group participants that the higher-level administrators could do more reach out to "managers and supervisors and ask them to let their employees know that it's okay for them to attend" wellness activities and encourage them to be flexible. One employee gave an example of how supervisors can be flexible: "because our office is actually usually busier during the lunch hour, it's when the people get off and come see us, [my supervisor] asked me if I wanted to take an hour in the morning to go [to the gym] instead of at lunch."
Other focus group participants (Employer E) shared that supervisors commonly perceive wellness program participation as a drain on productivity and took steps to discourage their workers from engaging in activities. Manufacturing workers at Employer D said managers are "too busy" and rarely discuss wellness activities or encourage participation in programs: "They don't know anything about it . . . they're everywhere else."

6.2.4. Make Full Use of Existing Resources and Relationships

All organizations in our case studies aim to leverage existing resources and build relationships, often with health plans, to expand offerings at little to no cost. Employer C, for example, implemented existing wellness programs that were advertised through the city government's website: a campaign to encourage employees to take the stairs and a fitness challenge requiring that participants track their steps. The organization worked with their health plan to offer onsite biometric screenings, seminars, and informational materials and improve their marketing and communication campaigns. This partnership has been crucial for allowing the company to offer a multi-component program on what they consider "a shoe-string budget."

Employer A, an educational institution, leveraged on-campus human capital by establishing mutually beneficial collaborations with different academic departments and programs/services and engaged students-in-training as service providers. Reliance on in-house resources allowed Employer A to offer individualized wellness activities that fit into the employees' busy schedules and to develop educational programs that showcase the expertise of its faculty members.

6.2.5. Continuously Evaluate and Improve Wellness Programs

Organizations from our case studies attempt to approach workplace wellness program with a continuous quality improvement attitude. Organizations improve programs by conducting needs assessments, improving feedback processes, and evaluating program success.

6.2.5.a. Wellness Needs Assessment

Employers use a number of different strategies to develop an understanding of the health risks and wellness needs of their workforce. These activities allow employers to design wellness programs that address their employees' specific risk factors and determine what interventions are of interest to employees. From our case studies, we learned that all employers conduct needs assessment with varying degrees of sophistication.

One employer (C) in our case study conducted rigorous needs assessments by examining employee- and organizational-level data and through consultation with third parties. Employer C partnered with its health plan to identify cost drivers among its employee population. This information was used to develop effective and relevant programs for employees. Organizational leaders decided that preventive care awareness would be the initial wellness priority, so wellness leaders researched medical standards for "appropriate care" and analyzed claims data to determine gaps in preventive screenings among their employee population. Further, the organization receives aggregate data from the results of the onsite biometric screening and online health questionnaire to inform wellness program development.

Other employers in our case studies assessed needs less formally—for instance, by consulting with individuals within the organization or contacting experts to identify health risks among the general population. Employer A developed a task force to identify major health and wellness-related areas of concern. The task force identified stress and work-life issues as important and chose a proactive approach trying to empower employees to change their habits, make better choices, and focus on health and wellness. Employer D reached out to public health experts at the CDC for advice on wellness program development, which prompted its decision to offer screenings coupled with educational classes to encourage individuals to manage their health risks.

Though all employers conducted needs assessments to some degree, wellness leaders stated that they implemented a number of wellness interventions simply based on the ease of implementation—that is, if educational materials or lifestyle management interventions were offered free through the health plan or external sources, employers would readily take advantage of them without formal planning.

6.2.5.b. Ongoing Feedback on Wellness Programs from Employees

Including employees in an ongoing feedback process, e.g., through surveys or the sharing of personal stories via email and personal conversation with program staff, can allow employers to further customize programs and develop benchmarks to monitor improvements. All employers from our case studies attempt to solicit feedback from staff with the goal of improving future wellness programming. However, employees often perceive their suggestions as undervalued and are not always engaged in the process.

According to one wellness program leader at Employer A, participants' feedback helps her understand the employee perspective and their satisfaction with program offerings. She gets "a lot of emails thanking [the program for] the massage therapy . . . and [for] anything that creates relaxation, such as free guided meditation sessions."

Employer C has a more formal approach for soliciting feedback: Wellness leaders ask employees to fill out a survey immediately after they complete their biometric screening, which has resulted in high response rates. Focus group participants reported mixed feelings as to whether their feedback is taken seriously. Some employees perceived their feedback as valuable: "They definitely want to know [our opinion] . . . every time they ask for feedback on a survey. Actually, I think they do a great job." Others expressed concern that their feedback wasn't taken into consideration: "the first time I provided feedback but then I didn't see anything change, so it's like, why am I wasting my time?"

Employer D administers a paper-based survey to manufacturing employees, since they are more difficult to reach, yet the majority of focus group participants said that they do not recall ever seeing a feedback survey, let alone completing it. The wellness champion responsible for compiling responses further supported this claim: "I know I collected [the feedback surveys] in the office, and there weren't that many that actually did it . . . there's not that many that offered suggestions."

6.2.5.c. Program Evaluation Is Uncommon But Viewed as Important

None of the employers in our case study conducted a formal evaluation of the impact of wellness programs. However, three of the five employers examined programs based on actionable performance measures, which include metrics on health outcomes (C, D) or cost and utilization (C, E). All five employers have some type of assessment—such as administering surveys to assess employee morale, self-reported changes in behavior, or trends in participation rates. We did not have access to the evaluation methodologies and therefore cannot verify the reported impacts. Evaluations described during interviews were often small scale and not methodologically rigorous.

Among employers in our case study, Employer C has conducted the most comprehensive outcome evaluation of its multifaceted wellness program:

> Through ongoing analyses of claims data and biometrics and a small-scale evaluation of a twelve-month nutrition program, the organization has been able to document positive impacts on employee health risks and behaviors and cost savings. The health plan estimates the savings derived from the wellness program by comparing the organization's healthcare cost against an industry benchmark, then leaders look at utilization patterns to compare findings. One organizational leader noted that savings align with measurable changes in care utilization patterns: "We noticed the savings since we've begun wellness initiatives . . . our emergency room visits have gone down, and we are above benchmark for all preventive care screenings."

Employer E conducted a one-time "Fitness Program Impact Study" to evaluate the impact of fitness leave on absenteeism, which estimated that every 20 hours of fitness leave was associated with a one-hour reduction in sick leave.[28]

Employer B found, through surveys, that nearly half of employees participate in a wellness program activity, and many employees report improved health behaviors, ranging from better management of

---

[28] Our contacts did not have access to the technical approach of this study, and we are therefore unable to verify the validity of this estimate.

stress to increased intake of fruits and vegetables. Although these data have not been linked to program participation, health care cost, or health outcomes data to measure program impact, they indicate that wellness programs are catching employees' attention.

Employer D asked wellness champions to track participation in a company-wide weight loss challenge, which, according to focus group participants, is the best-known wellness activity at the organization. Ten percent of the employee population (n = 629) participate in this weight loss program, and nearly a quarter of those participating (n = 140) are employed in the corporate headquarters. By documenting participation rates, wellness leaders realize that they need to reevaluate their recruitment strategy to improve employee engagement, particularly among workers in the manufacturing plants, and are looking to third-party vendors for strategic advice.

Chapter 7: Conclusions

Our project combined a literature review, a national survey of employers, case studies of workplace wellness programs, and statistical analyses of the CCA database to assess current use of workplace wellness programs in the United States, estimate the effect of programs on employee health and health care costs, and evaluate the role of incentives for program engagement. We find that wellness programs have become a common workplace benefit and that employers remain optimistic about their impact. Well-executed programs appear to improve employee health meaningfully, whereas significant reductions in health care cost may take time to materialize. As employee engagement in programs remains limited, employers are commonly using incentives tied to participation in screening activities and programs and occasionally to achieving health-related standards. Although participation incentives appear to be effective, intended and unintended effects of incentives for health-related standards need to be studied further.

7.1. Wellness Benefits and Program Uptake Among Employers

Our study shows that workplace wellness programs have emerged as a common employer-sponsored benefit that is now available at about half of U.S. employers with 50 or more employees, which employ three-quarters of the U.S. workforce employed at firms and organizations of that size. Larger employers are more likely than small employers to offer a wellness program and also tend to offer programs with a variety of options. Most employers are committed to long-term support of wellness programs, as they regard them as a viable strategy to contain health care costs, thereby ensuring the affordability of health coverage. In spite of their popularity at workplace, the impact of wellness programs is rarely formally evaluated by employers.

We find that a clear picture is emerging about how employers today offer workplace wellness benefits to their employees. Four components form a typical wellness strategy:

(1) **Wellness programs,** which include
   a. *Screening activities,* such as HRAs, clinical screening (e.g., blood pressure measurement)
   b. *Preventive interventions,* such as lifestyle management (e.g., smoking cessation) and disease management (e.g., diabetes management) to address health risks and prevent exacerbation

106

      c. *Health promotion benefits,* such as on-site vaccinations and healthy food options that are accessible to all employees regardless of existing health risks

(2) **Other health and well-being-related benefits***,* such as EAPs

(3) Changes in **benefit design** to encourage healthy behaviors

      a. *Incentives* as part of health coverage (e.g., variation in employees' share of health plan premiums based on smoking status)

      b. *Incentives* offered directly by an employer (e.g., cash payments for fitness program participants)

(4) **Structural changes** to the worksite that promote healthy behaviors, such as installation of walkways on campus to promote walking.

(5) **Contextual changes** to promote program effect, such as leadership support and changes to corporate culture and policies.

Employer-based wellness programs focus on risk factors for metabolic, cardiovascular, and pulmonary diseases, as they are the most prevalent chronic conditions in the working-age population, but offer a variety of interventions that are tailored to specific workplace environments, such as stress reduction and back pain programs.

7.2. Program Impact

Consistent with prior research, we find that lifestyle management programs as part of workplace wellness can reduce risk factors, such as smoking, and increase healthy behaviors, such as exercise. We find that these effects are sustainable over time and clinically meaningful. This result is of critical importance, as it confirms that workplace wellness programs can help contain the current epidemic of lifestyle-related diseases, the main driver of premature morbidity and mortality in the United States.

Our estimates of wellness program impact on health care costs are lower than most results reported in the literature, but we caution that our approach estimated the isolated impact of lifestyle management interventions, whereas a majority of published studies captured the overall effect of an employer's approach to health and wellness. Although we do not detect statistically significant decreases in cost and use of emergency department and hospital care, the trends in health care costs and use of high-cost care for program participants and nonparticipants diverge over time. Therefore, there is reason to believe that reduction in direct medical costs would materialize if employees continued to participate in a wellness program. Lacking access to proprietary information on program cost, we could not estimate the program effect on overall cost of coverage directly but, judging by published data, the programs would become cost-neutral after five years.

Our case studies and the review of the literature also highlight a number of factors that may affect wellness program success in the workplace. Effective communication with employees about program goals and benefits, accessibility and alignment with employee needs, leadership support, creative use of resources, and continuous program improvement all appear to be factors that can improve employee health and increase the effectiveness of worksite wellness programs, even though their actual impact on effectiveness and cost-effectiveness of programs still needs to be evaluated.

7.3. Role of Incentives

Employers regard limited employee engagement as an important obstacle to program success, and data from the RAND Employer Survey confirm that rates of employee participation in screening and management programs remain low. To promote program uptake, employers offer incentives directly or through their group health plans, as the RAND Employer Survey and other surveys suggest. Data from the CCA database show that incentives of over $5 per year appear effective in getting employees to complete an HRA. We cannot assess the impact of incentives above $100 per year, as this was the maximum amount used by the employers in the CCA database. Anecdotally, larger incentives can be effective, such as the $50 *per week* that Employer D in our case studies used, to achieve almost 100 percent participation in onsite clinical screenings. Modest incentives also seem to increase participation in and impact of lifestyle management programs.

An important policy question is whether "high-powered" incentives that link amounts of 20 percent or more of the cost of individual coverage to attainment of health goals or alternative standards should be permitted or even promoted. On one hand, such incentives might encourage employees to fundamentally change health-related behaviors; on the other, they might place a disproportionate burden on lower-paid workers, as they tend to have more health risk factors.

None of the employers in the CCA database used incentives of any size linked to attaining personal health goals. We were therefore not able to empirically test their impact on health status, cost of

108

coverage, and unintended consequences, but several findings of our study can, nonetheless, inform policy deliberations on this question.

First, the use of incentives tied to health standards remains uncommon. The RAND Employer Survey suggests that nationally, only 10 percent of employers with 50 or more employees use any such incentives, and only 7 percent link the incentives to the premiums for health coverage. The average maximum incentive amount for these employers was less than 10 percent of the total annual cost of coverage, far from the 20 percent regulatory threshold. The one health risk factor for which results-based incentives are more common and involve higher amounts is smoking, as suggested by both the RAND Employer Survey and our case studies.

Our statistical analyses show a small effect of participation incentives up to $200, which is the range reported in our data, on weight, smoking, and exercise. On the positive side, employers in our case studies do not appear to use incentive schemes as a tool to simply shift cost to employees but strongly attempt to support employees in achieving their targets. As an executive at one case study employer stated: "If I just wanted to increase cost sharing, I could just do that without a complicated incentive scheme."

At the same time, case study findings imply that the risk of unintended consequences is real. We consistently observed that shift, part-time, and off-site employees could not take full advantage of their employer's program, because of limited flexibility in their schedules, remote location, and less understanding of program goals and benefits. Thus, the combination of the higher prevalence of health risk factors and more limited access to interventions that can ameliorate those risks may lead to a differential shifting of cost to such employees, when substantial incentives are tied to lowering health risks. In developing policy and making decisions, this possible unintended effect should be weighed against the potential beneficial consequences of increased employee participation in programs in response to strong incentives.

7.4. Future Research
This project represents the most comprehensive analysis of worksite wellness programs to date and has clearly contributed to an improved understanding of current program participation, program impact, and the role of incentives. Our findings highlight priority areas for future research.

7.4.1. Long-Term Impact of Wellness Programs

Our study was able to detect statistically significant and clinically meaningful effects of wellness programs on health risk factors after examining six years of CCA data. Given the long latency between health risks and the development of manifest chronic disease, however, a much longer follow-up period will be required to fully capture the effect of worksite wellness programs on health outcomes and cost. Additionally, a broader sample could possibly allow generalization of results to a larger population of employers.

7.4.2. Impact on a Broader Range of Measures

We analyzed the impact of workplace wellness programs on health risks and health care use. Future studies should look at a broader range of outcomes, in particular, work-related outcomes and health-related quality of life. Work-related outcomes, such as absenteeism, productivity, and retention, are of critical importance to employers as they directly affect business performance. Therefore, understanding the effect of wellness programs on those outcomes will guide employers' decisions on investment in the health of their workforce. Determining impact on quality of life measures can inform the broader policy question on welfare implications of wellness programs.

7.4.3. Unpacking the Black Box: Contextual Factors That Modify Program Effects

As with any complex intervention, contextual factors will influence the effectiveness and cost-effectiveness of workplace wellness interventions. In other words, a program design might work well for a particular employer but not in a different context. Different workforces might require different approaches to program design and execution. Our current study provides a high-level analysis of overall program impact, but it did not have the sample size and variation in program types and employer to explore such questions.

Program Design and Delivery

A more granular examination of different program components would provide valuable insights into determinants of program success. For example, such analyses could compare the differential effects of modalities for program delivery (e.g., telephone, Internet, and in-person). They could investigate a possible dose-response relationship between program interactions and results, i.e., whether more contacts are more effective and cost-effective and whether there are increasing and decreasing effects of higher intensity. They could also compare the relative effect of individual-level and workforce-level interventions. Understanding differences between the designs of different programs could help to identify success factors and potential pitfalls to avoid to improve program development. Conducting such studies would require data from a much larger and more diverse sample than ours to have the statistical power and the variation to detect differential impact of particular program features.

Employer Factors

Our literature review and case studies identified a variety of considerations for the successful implementation of worksite wellness programs, such as leadership support and communication. It is plausible to expect that taking these factors into account will improve program impact. However, before promoting them as best practice, it would be prudent to determine how they affect employee participation and health outcomes in future studies and to quantify their relative contribution. Similarly, such employer characteristics as workplace culture might modify the effect of wellness programs. Understanding the role of such modifying factors would require data from a large sample of employers with differences in program implementation and characteristics to compare and contrast. Of particular interest would be data from smaller employers (i.e., those with less 50 employees), as they account for a large share of the workforce but may have limited resources to devote to wellness programs.

Employee Characteristics

The ultimate goal of wellness interventions is to change health-related behaviors and self-management of risk factors and manifest diseases. To achieve this goal, programs need to first engage employees and then deliver an intervention that is audience-appropriate and effective. As evident from the low rate of program uptake in our study, more research into employee engagement is clearly needed. We need to understand better how employee demographic characteristics (such as age and gender), psychological states (such as self-efficacy), and educational attainment (such as health literacy) drive decisions about program uptake and how those factors interact with financial incentives. Such information would help to improve program outreach and to make programs more inclusive for employees with diverse backgrounds. The same consideration holds true for program delivery: We need to understand better how different employees respond to different modalities, content, and intensity to develop audience-appropriate and effective interventions.

7.4.4. Effects of Financial Incentives

We find that financial incentives are commonly used to encourage participation in screening activities and wellness interventions but are less frequently tied to health standards. In particular, high-powered incentives that tie a substantial proportion of the cost of coverage to specific health standards remain rare. Our database for the statistical analyses did not contain employers with health-contingent programs, and we were unable to assess intended and unintended effects of such programs directly. As incentives tied to health standards in general and high-powered incentives are not commonly used, it will remain difficult to attempt to study them with observational studies such as ours. Rather, a prospective study that seeks to deliberately recruit employers with such incentives or even an experimental study that introduces different incentive levels under controlled conditions may be required. In addition, there is limited information of the differential impact of different incentive types. For example, rewards may have a different effect than penalties and premium reductions may have a different effect than cash payments. These questions need to be studied further to help optimize use of incentives.

Appendix A: Employer Survey Sampling Methods

Sample Stratification

We classified industry by the four main categories of the 2007 North America Industry Classification System (NAICS), as shown in Table A1. The NAICS is considered a standard and well-established classification system. We determined that the classification into four groups provides sufficient granularity, because Categories 1 and 2 both include blue-collar industries, but Category 1 is more characterized by strenuous manual labor, implying a different workforce composition and different health risks. Categories 3 and 4 predominantly consist of white-collar workers, but the constraints and opportunities to offer wellness programs are different in the public compared to the private service sector.

Table A1: Industry Categories Used for Sampling

2007 NAICS	Industry Description	Industry Category
11	Agriculture, Forestry, Fishing and Hunting	
21	Mining, Quarrying, and Oil and Gas Extraction	
22	Utilities	Category 1
23	Construction	
31-33	Manufacturing	
42	Wholesale Trade	
44-45	Retail Trade	Category 2
48-49	Transportation and Warehousing	
51	Information	
52	Finance and Insurance	
53	Real Estate and Rental and Leasing	
54	Professional, Scientific, and Technical Services	
55	Management of Companies and Enterprises	
56	Administrative and Support and Waste Management and Remediation Services	Category 3
61	Educational Services	
62	Health Care and Social Assistance	
71	Arts, Entertainment, and Recreation	
72	Accommodation and Food Services	
81	Other Services (except Public Administration)	
92	Federal governments - Public Administration	
92	State governments - Public Administration	Category 4
92	Local governments - Public Administration	

SOURCE: U.S. Census Bureau NAICS.

We decided to categorize firm size by number of employees and form five categories:

- ≥ 50 and ≤ 100 workers
- > 100 and ≤ 1000 workers
- $> 1,000$ and $\leq 10,000$ workers
- $> 10,000$ and $\leq 50,000$ workers
- $> 50,000$ workers

First, we excluded employers with fewer than 50 workers, because they are subject to different regulations. For example, the Affordable Care Act exempts them from penalties if they do not offer health insurance coverage, and most states consider them part of the small group market. They typically have a different range of health-related benefits, as the small group market has less sophisticated insurance products and lower coverage rates. Use of wellness programs tends to be lower and customization of programs rare.

Although the same holds true for firms with 50–100 employees, they are subject to different regulations, as they are guaranteed to be able to offer health insurance coverage on the newly created health insurance exchanges by 2016.

Firms with 100–1,000 staff begin to offer wellness programs to a greater extent but typically rely on solutions offered by their health insurance carriers. Firms with 1,000 to 10,000 employees have the scale to customize wellness programs with respect to program scope, content, and strategies to increase enrollment. Above 1,000 staff, companies also begin to self-insure. Very large employers with more than 10,000 workers are in a position to develop their own programs and participation strategies, with the most sophisticated and mature programs seen in firms with more than 50,000 staff.

Sample Allocation

Combining four industry categories with five categories for firm size yields 20 sampling strata, with on average 150 draws based on our starting sample of 3,000 firms, allowing for a reasonable cell size. The population sizes in each of our 20 strata are substantially different. For example, there are far fewer firms with more than 50,000 employees and far more firms in the service sector. Consequently, we cannot allocate the 3,000 starting firms equally to each stratum, if we want to generate valid estimates.

There are different algorithms to allocate the available sample to the strata, and the choice of the best algorithm is driven by two competing goals:

(1) to produce a precise estimate for the overall prevalence[29] of program offering, as expressed by a low margin of error for the overall prevalence estimate

(2) to enable credible comparisons between employers in different employment size or industry categories, as expressed by a low minimal detectable difference between two categories.

The optimal sample allocation algorithm for one goal might not be optimal for the other. Thus, we simulated five different allocation scenarios to identify an algorithm that allows for comparisons between our categories for industry and firm size but maintains the precision of the overall prevalence estimate.

(1) Allocating sampling units in proportion to the stratum population.

That is, strata with a larger number of employers (e.g., strata with 50100 workers per employer or industry category 3 will be assigned a proportionately larger share of the 3,000 sampling units.

(2) Maximizing the effective sample size for each stratum without weighting.

The purpose of maximizing the effective sample size for each stratum is to get homogeneous, effective sample sizes for each of the 20 sampling strata. Effective sample size is the number of sampling units in a stratum adjusted by the finite population correction factor,[30] which accounts for the fact that the sample does not come from an infinitely large population. To implement this algorithm, we wrote a computer program to allocate the sampling units. The program first allocates one sampling unit to each of the 20 strata and then assigns the next unit to the cell with the smallest effective sample size. The process is repeated until all the 3,000 sampling units are assigned.

(3) Maximizing the effective sample size for each stratum, weighted by the estimated variance of prevalence.

---

[29] We discuss the sample allocation decisions using overall wellness program prevalence as an example, but the same considerations apply to other estimates that will be generated in the study, such as prevalence of use of incentives.
[30] Finite population correction is used to adjust for the fact that our sample is drawn without replacement from a population with a finite size, whereas statistical inferences are based on the premise that samples are drawn from an infinitely large population.

This is Algorithm (2), except that strata with a larger variance of overall prevalence, estimated according to KFF/HRET (2010), will receive a larger proportion of the 3,000 sampling units. The rationale is that a greater number of sampling units allocated to strata with greater variance will produce more precise estimates for these strata and thus a more precise overall program offering rate.

(4) Maximizing the effective sample size for each stratum, weighted by employment size. This algorithm maximizes the effective sample size for each stratum, but strata with larger companies (e.g., strata with 10,000–50,000 workers per employer) will receive a larger proportion of the 3,000 sampling units. Because larger firms are more likely to offer a multi-component programs and tailor it to the needs of their employees, assigning more sampling units to strata with larger companies will oversample the employers with more comprehensive programs than would be the case with Algorithm (2). As a result, this approach will enrich the type of programs and/or incentives used in the final sample.

(5) Maximizing the effective sample size for each stratum, weighted by the variance and employment size simultaneously. A combination of Algorithms (3) and (4), it gives more weight to strata with either a larger variance in prevalence or to those with larger employment size.

The results of the simulations are presented in Table A2. The results show that maximizing the effective sample size without weighting (Algorithm 2) performs best in balancing our two goals of maximizing overall precision while allowing discrimination between size and industry categories. Based on power calculations that assume a response rate of 35 percent, the final estimate of the overall prevalence of program offering will have a margin of error of 5 percentage points, based on a sample of 3,000 employers (Table A2). We have 80 percent power to detect a 12 percentage point difference between Industry Category 1 (agriculture, mining, construction, and manufacturing) and Category 4 (governments), using a two-sided test and a significance level of 5 percent. Similarly, the minimum detectable difference between employer size category of 50–100 and 10,001–50,000 is 12.59 percentage points. When the response rate is 45 percent, the margin of error of the overall rate is 4.5 percentage points, and the minimum detectable difference across industries or employment size categories is about 11 percentage points.

116

Table A2: Sample Size Considerations

Response Rate	Sampling Units Allocation Algorithm	Marginal Error of the Overall Prevalence	Minimum Detectable Prevalence Difference Between Industry Category 1 and Category 4[a]	Minimum Detectable Prevalence Difference Between Employment Size 50–100 vs. 10,001–50,000 Categories[a]
35%	Proportional to Stratum Population	3.02	17.58	42.33
	Maximizing Stratum-specific Effective Sample Size	5.15	12.25	12.59
	Maximizing Stratum-specific Effective Sample Size, Weighted by Estimated Variance of Prevalence	9.44	16.53	17.35
	Maximizing Stratum-specific Effective Sample Size, Weighted by Employment Size	27.71	59.22	51.08
	Maximizing Stratum-specific Effective Sample Size, Weighted by Variance and Employment Size	58.50	87.43	100.00
45%	Proportional to Stratum Population	2.67	15.52	37.59
	Maximizing Stratum-specific Effective Sample Size	4.54	10.80	11.10
	Maximizing Stratum-specific Effective Sample Size, Weighted by Estimated Variance of Prevalence	8.32	14.58	15.31
	Maximizing Stratum-specific Effective Sample Size, Weighted by Employment Size	24.44	52.23	45.05
	Maximizing Stratum-specific Effective Sample Size, Weighted by Variance and Employment Size	51.60	77.11	94.92

[a] In percentage points; with 80 percent power and a significance level of 5 percent; based on a two-sided test and a sample of 3,000 employers.

Allocating samples proportionally to the size of each stratum does produce a small margin of error, about 3 percentage points. However, it allocates only a very small number of units for some strata, especially those with a large number of employees. For example, all strata with more than 10,000 workers have fewer than five units, which does not allow us to make valid comparisons for these

117

categories because of imprecise estimates. The minimum detectable prevalence difference between the strata with 50–100 workers and that with 10,001–50,000 is 42 percentage points, assuming a response rate of 35 percent (Table A2). A similar problem arises when weighted by employment size, where strata with small employment receive only five units. When weighted by the variance of prevalence, strata with larger variance receive more units than those with smaller variance, but overall, this algorithm does not outperform the one without weighting. Therefore, we used the results from Algorithm (2) that maximizes the effective sample size for each stratum without weighting. Table A3 shows the resulting allocation.

Table A3: Sample Allocation Results

Employment Size	Industries	2007 NAICS	Stratum Population	Sample Allocation	Effective Sample Size
01: 50-100	Cat1	11-33	44,003	195	196
01: 50-100	Cat2	42-49	32,141	195	196
01: 50-100	Cat3	51-81	112,244	196	196
01: 50-100	Cat4	92	5,487	189	196
02: 101-1000	Cat1	11-33	30,784	195	196
02: 101-1000	Cat2	42-49	17,582	194	196
02: 101-1000	Cat3	51-81	70,028	196	197
02: 101-1000	Cat4	92	6,396	190	196
03: 1001-10,000	Cat1	11-33	4,249	187	196
03: 1001-10,000	Cat2	42-49	1,901	178	196
03: 1001-10,000	Cat3	51-81	9,666	192	196
03: 1001-10,000	Cat4	92	1,081	166	196
04: 10,001-50,000	Cat1	11-33	467	139	197
04: 10,001-50,000	Cat2	42-49	317	122	198
04: 10,001-50,000	Cat3	51-81	922	162	196
04: 10,001-50,000	Cat4	92	138	82	201
05: 50,001+	Cat1	11-33	75	55	204
05: 50,001+	Cat2	42-49	63	48	198
05: 50,001+	Cat3	51-81	138	82	201
05: 50,001+	Cat4	92	44	37	227
Total			337,726	3,000	3,974

SOURCE: Based on KFF/HRET (2010).

Response Rates and Sampling Weights

As illustrated in Table A4, the overall response rate was 19 percent. Employers with an employment size between 101 and 1,000 and governments had the largest response rates (24 percent and 29 percent,

Table A4: Employer Survey Response Rates, by Size of Employer and Industry Response Rate

Employment Size	Rate
50-100	20%
101-1000	24%
1001-10,000	17%
10,001-50,000	18%
50,001+	13%
Industry	
Heavy industry	15%
Trade	18%
Services	18%
Government	29%
Total	19%

NOTE: Response rate = completed responses/(companies contacted – ineligible companies).

respectively). The response rates and sampling weights for each stratum are presented in Table A5. Response rates differed across sampling strata, ranging from 6 percent among employers with more than 50,000 employees and in Industry Category 1 (e.g., agriculture and manufacturing) to 34 percent among government agencies with an employment size between 101 and 1,000.

119

Table A5: Employer Survey Response Rates and Sampling Weights, by Sampling Strata

Employment Size	Industries	Adjusted Stratum Population[a]	Response Rate	Sampling Weight
01: 50-100	Cat1	39,490	17%	1234.1
01: 50-100	Cat2	29,669	22%	674.3
01: 50-100	Cat3	99,645	13%	3985.8
01: 50-100	Cat4	5,487	28%	101.6
02: 101-1000	Cat1	28,100	16%	936.7
02: 101-1000	Cat2	17,310	23%	360.6
02: 101-1000	Cat3	65,026	21%	1512.2
02: 101-1000	Cat4	6,396	34%	96.9
03: 1001-10,000	Cat1	4,090	13%	157.3
03: 1001-10,000	Cat2	1,880	12%	85.4
03: 1001-10,000	Cat3	9,414	18%	261.5
03: 1001-10,000	Cat4	1,081	25%	25.7
04: 10,001-50,000	Cat1	464	18%	17.8
04: 10,001-50,000	Cat2	301	10%	25.1
04: 10,001-50,000	Cat3	911	17%	32.5
04: 10,001-50,000	Cat4	138	33%	5.1
05: 50,001+	Cat1	74	6%	24.5
05: 50,001+	Cat2	62	11%	12.3
05: 50,001+	Cat3	135	17%	9.6
05: 50,001+	Cat4	42	16%	6.9

[a] Adjusted by the proportion of ineligible employers that did not exist at the time of survey because they went out of business or merged.

Table A6: Characteristics of Employer Survey Nonrespondents and Respondents

Characteristics	Nonrespondent (%)	Respondent (%)
Employer size[**]		
50 to 100	26.0	26.3
101 to 1,000	25.0	31.7
1,001 to 10,000	24.7	21.4
10,001 to 50,000	16.6	15.8
> 50,000	7.7	4.8
Industry [**]		
Heavy industry	27.4	19.9
Trade	25.7	22.2
Services	28.3	24.8
Government	18.6	33.1
Region[**]		
Northeast	22.3	17.7
Midwest	23.4	28.0
South	35.3	32.6
West	18.1	21.6
Subsidiary (%)[**]	34.4	22.8
Limited to nongovernment entities		
Revenue, in millions (SD)	$3,584 ($17,705)	$2,687 ($9,450)
Years in business (SD)[*]	44.0 (37.3)	48.4 (38.1)
Women owned (%)	3.6	2.3
Minority owned (%)	3.2	3.3

$*p < 0.05$; $** p < 0.01$.

121

Appendix B: CCA Data Analysis Methods

Analytic Sample

To obtain our analytic sample, we applied a number of inclusion and exclusion criteria. As shown in Table B1, we restricted the sample to active full-time employees between the ages of 18 and 64 about whom the database has at least one full year of data. We excluded employee years associated with enrollment in health maintenance organizations (HMO) or other capitated health insurance plans for two reasons. First, medical or prescriptions claims for these plan types are likely to be incomplete, and second, these plan types are more likely to offer programs that resemble those in typical employer-based wellness programs. We excluded employee years during which the employee was pregnant, since this might have an impact on health behaviors, health outcomes, medical costs, and health care use.

For each research question, specific exclusion criteria were applied to create an appropriate analytic subsample. For example, to look at the effect of incentives on health outcomes, we restricted the sample to employees who have at least two consecutive years of health outcomes data for the outcome in question. As shown in Table B1, the availability of health outcome and behavior data was limited across the seven employers.

After applying all of our additional criteria, the majority of our analyses used analytic subsamples composed of data from four (referred to as Employers 1, 2, 3, and 4) of the seven employers given to us for analysis from the Data Aggregation Project. Below, we briefly describe the key characteristics of these four employers, as well as sample sizes following each inclusion and exclusion criteria.

The overall characteristics of the four employers with data meeting the requirements for most of our analyses are shown in Table B2. Three of the four employers had geographic reach across most regions of the United States. The employers had somewhat large differences in the proportion of female employees, as well as in the proportion of employees who work full-time. Compensation also differed across employers, with Employer 4 having an average compensation roughly double that of Employer 2.

An important factor that limited our analytic subsamples was length of employee tenure, meaning the number of complete years of data. Employee tenure ranged from one year to six years. For example, employees with only one year of data could not be used for most analyses, as our main analytic

122

Table B1: Creation of an Analytic Sample from the Data Aggregation Project Secondary Data

Inclusion Criteria	Number of EmployeeYears	Number of Unique Employees	Number of Employers
1. Aged 18–64	1,793,884	567,506	7
2. One or more full-year enrollment	1,351,478	428,974	7
3. Active full-time	1,206,327	382,459	7
4. Not enrolled in HMO	1,039,136	327,024	7
5. With complete claims data	977,100	292,792	6
6. Not pregnant during data year	951,112	287,694	6
Additional criteria for analytic subsamples			
HRA data available	611,862	232,037	6
Program participation data available	615,770	173,382	4
BMI data available	306,950	149,844	6
Total cholesterol data available	104,086	66,301	6
Exercise data available	109,487	58,858	3
Smoking status data available	111,912	61,486	4

SOURCE: RAND analysis of health plan claims and screening and wellness program data in the CCA database.
NOTE: Data on high-density lipoprotein and low-density lipoprotein are not complete.

Table B2: Characteristics of Employers in the CCA Data Analytic Sample

	Employer 1	Employer 2	Employer 3	Employer 4
Primary Industry	Manufacturing	Accommodation/Services	Educational Services	Manufacturing
Total employees (no.)	28,341	7,569	39,272	136,824
Average compensation ($ 1000s)[a]	50–75	25–50	50–75	75–100
Part-time employees (%)	1.9	86.2	19.2	0.6
Female (%)	12.5	52.2	59.9	29.5
Region of employment (%)				
Northeast	20.6	7.0	0.8	3.4
North central	10.6	19.3	97.1	14.4
South	44.4	59.9	1.1	11.5
West	24.3	13.7	0.8	70.6
Unknown	0.0	0	0.3	0.1

SOURCE: RAND analysis of health plan claims and screening and wellness program data in the CCA database.
[a] Nonexecutive full-time employees

strategies required being able to see changes across time for individual employees. Across the four employers in most of our analyses, more than half of employees had a tenure of at least three years, suggesting moderate employee turnover overall.

Figure B1 shows the number of program participants among the four employers by program eligibility and program type. Approximately two-thirds to three-quarters of program participants were eligible for the program based on their HRA.

For example, employees are typically eligible to join a weight control program if they are overweight or obese. In addition, employers commonly permit employees to participate in certain programs, even if they do not meet formal eligibility requirements but only want to improve their health. For example, employees with normal weight may be able to enroll in a nutritional counseling program to learn about healthier food options. Of note, eligibility as defined by program vendors varies, because employers used different vendors and the eligibility criteria may be different.

Figure B1: Wellness Program Participation, by Employee Program Eligibility Status and Program Type

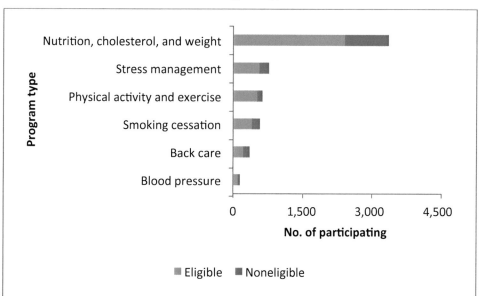

SOURCE: RAND analysis of health plan claims and screening and wellness program data in the CCA database.
NOTES: Data shown are for 2009 only. Eligibility is based on HRA results, but employers permit employees who do not meet formal eligibility criteria to participate in selected programs. Employer 4 data were missing the program eligibility variable, and we assumed that all employees were eligible for the program(s) for which they had participation records.

124

Multivariate Analysis for the Impact of Program Participation

This multivariate analysis quantifies the impact of program participation on health behaviors, health outcomes, medical cost, and health care use. As described above, our analytic strategy was to compare program participants to nonparticipants. But simply using nonparticipants as the comparison group may yield biased estimates, because nonparticipants may be different from participants in observed and unobserved dimensions. To address this issue, we adopted a two-step approach:

(1) identifying a valid comparison group using propensity score matching

(2) performing longitudinal regression analysis using the matched pairs from Step (1).

In Step (1), we used propensity score matching to identify comparison members who are similar to program participants in observed characteristics at baseline. First, we constructed a propensity regression using the information available in a baseline year when both groups did not participate in a program and predicted a propensity score for each employee. The propensity regression takes the following form:

$$\text{Logit}(p) = \beta_0 + X\beta_1 + E\beta_2 + T\beta_3 \qquad\qquad \text{Equation (i)}$$

where p is the propensity of participating in any wellness program in the years after the baseline year, X is a vector of employee characteristics, E is a vector of employer indicators, and T is a vector of year indicators. Employee characteristics include employee age in ten-year intervals, gender, number of years in the data (employee tenure), enrollment in a capitated health plan, region (Northeast, Midwest, South, and West), being a union member, indicators of Charlson comorbidities, baseline per-member per-month medical cost, baseline inpatient admissions, and baseline emergency department visits.

We then used a one-to-one matching algorithm to match participants to similar nonparticipants based on their propensity of participation, stratified by employer and the baseline year. After matching, all the observed characteristics at baseline were balanced between participants and nonparticipants based on a significance level of 5 percent. In the matching process, we did not use the eligibility as defined by program vendors, because employers used different vendors and the eligibility criteria may be different. In addition, many employees participated in a program regardless of their eligibility status.

In Step (2), we conducted longitudinal regression analysis to account for the unobserved employee characteristics using employee-level fixed effects. The longitudinal analysis generated impact estimates for multiple-year program participation, varying from one year to five years. Also, we explored whether program effectiveness differs across calendar years, employers, and regions. Because program participation data were available for only a small number of, we were not able to examine whether the effectiveness varies across different industries. The longitudinal regression takes the following form:

$$D_{it} = \alpha_i + P_{it}\beta_1 + X_{it}\beta_2 + T\beta_3 + \varepsilon_{it} \qquad \text{Equation (ii)}$$

where D is the annualized difference between the outcome of interest in year *t* and baseline for employee *i*, α_i is employee fixed effect, P_{it} is a vector of participation indicators, X_{it} is a vector of time varying employee characteristics, T is a vector of year indicators, and ε_{it} is the error term.

Participation indicators include participation status in the current year, prior year, two years ago, three years ago, and four years ago. A participation indicator in other programs was added when we examined a specific program, e.g., cholesterol control. Employee characteristics include employee age in ten-year intervals, enrollment in a capitated health plan, region indicators, being a union member, and indicators of Charlson comorbidities. Note that employer indicators were not included because of employee fixed effect. Robust standard errors were used for all longitudinal analysis. The coefficient estimates of program participation indicators are difference in differences estimates.

For the analysis of smoking status, we required that all employees be smokers at baseline, since only smokers are eligible for a smoking cessation program. In other words, we matched smokers who participated in a smoking cessation program at least once in the years following baseline with smokers who did not participate in such a program in the years following baseline.

Our analytic strategies addressed two main challenges to validity of such observational analyses:

(1) Selection bias, which refers to the fact that participants may be better motivated for improving health than nonparticipants. Thus, a simple comparison of participants to nonparticipants may result in an overestimation of program impact. First, our propensity score matching method ensures the comparability of two groups in their observed characteristics. Second, our longitudinal regression analysis controlled for unobserved employee characteristics that are not

available in our data but remain constant over time. In technical language, it is an individual-level fixed effect in a longitudinal analysis.

(2) Regression to the mean, which refers to the fact that employees with high medical costs at baseline may have lower medical costs in subsequent years, i.e., when they have enrolled in the program. The opposite is true for members with low costs at baseline. This bias may confound estimates of program impacts. Our propensity score matching ensured that participants and nonparticipants were similar at baseline.

In addition to the propensity score matching approach, we used propensity score as weights in the longitudinal analysis that included all participants and nonparticipants. Using propensity score weighting generated similar results and failed to change the conclusions.

Success in Propensity Score Matching

The success rate is defined as the proportion of program participants that can be matched to a statistically similar nonparticipant. As shown in Table B3, the success rate in propensity score matching is greater than 90 percent for all the outcome of interest except BMI (79 percent). This might be due to self-selection into a weight control program. In other words, program participants are more likely to have a larger BMI and, compared to other outcomes of interest, it was more difficult to find a nonparticipant with a similar BMI to that of a participant. After matching, all the covariates are balanced at the 5 percent significance level.

Table B3: Success in Propensity Score Matching

Outcome of Interest	Program Participants	Nonparticipants	Matched Pairs	Success Rate	Variables Not Balanced After Matching[a]
Exercise	2,433	13,627	2,303	94.66%	None
Smoking	772	2,797	746	96.63%	None
BMI	4,978	60,043	3,924	78.83%	None
Total cholesterol	1,481	18,151	1,341	90.55%	None
Cost and utilizations	12,734	128,356	12,127	95.23%	None

[a]Unbalanced if p < 0.05.

Simulation Analyses to Demonstrate Cumulative Program Effects

Our regression analyses yield estimates for program effects in each program year, but workplace wellness programs are multiyear interventions that are expected to achieve benefits over time, as they change health-related behaviors and reduce risk factors. We therefore sought to devise an intuitive way to estimate and present cumulative program effects based on the regression results.

We took a hypothetical cohort of employees who are representative of the estimation sample. We used this cohort to simulate outcomes as if they participated in the program (intervention cohort); similarly, we used the same cohort to simulate outcomes as if they did not participate (comparison cohort). We then applied program effects derived from regressions, where program participation would have an effect starting in the first year of participation but also in the subsequent years. For example, educating an overweight employee about healthy eating and exercise would help to reduce his or her weight in the first year of program participation and also have an effect in subsequent years because of lasting behavior change. We tested whether impacts varied over time by adding interaction terms between participation indicators and year indicators and adjusted simulations accordingly if program effectiveness varied across calendar years. We also accounted for secular trends that would lead to changes in outcomes for the intervention and comparison cohorts alike.

As an example, our simulation starts at the baseline level for average weight in both cohorts, reflects secular changes for both cohorts over time, and captures both the immediate effect of program participation and its enduring effect because of lasting behavior change.

Using the estimated effects of program participation from the longitudinal regressions, we obtained the effect of current year participation on the outcomes for the current year and the subsequent years.

The coefficients of year indicators capture the secular trends in the outcome of interest. We then simulated a homogeneous cohort of employees who have the average employee characteristics in the estimation sample and participate in a program consecutively during a five-year period (2006–2010) with 2005 as the baseline year (intervention cohort). The average employee characteristics were set at the mean level of the estimation sample, including the baseline outcomes. We simulated the same cohort of employees who do not participate in the program during the same time period (comparison cohort). The simulated outcomes contain two components: the secular trends and the program effect estimates, but the difference in the outcomes between two cohorts represents program effect estimates only.

Simulated outcome = Baseline outcome + Secular trend + Program effects

In the model specifications, we considered both the potential lag effects of program participation and the differential effects of participation over time. As illustrated in Equation (iii), coefficients E_t, E_{t-1}, E_{t-3}, and E_{t-4} represent the effects of participation in the current year, the prior year, two years ago, three years ago, and four years ago, respectively. In addition, differential effects across calendar years are represented by coefficients (γ) of the interaction terms between program participation (P) and calendar years (T). Given that our data cover the years 2005–2010, some interactions between lag program effects apply to only some of the calendar years. For example, participation two years ago only applies to 2008 and beyond, and the interaction with calendar year 2007 is not applicable.

$$
\begin{aligned}
D_{it} = &\; \alpha_i + E_t P_{it} + E_{t-1} P_{i(t-1)} + E_{t-2} P_{i(t-2)} + E_{t-3} P_{i(t-3)} + E_{t-4} P_{i(t-4)} \\
&+ \beta_{11} T_{2007} + \beta_{12} T_{2008} + \beta_{13} T_{2009} + \beta_{14} T_{2010} \\
&+ \gamma_{t1} P_{it}{}^* T_{2007} + \gamma_{t2} P_{it}{}^* T_{2008} + \gamma_{t3} P_{it}{}^* T_{2009} + \gamma_{t4} P_{it}{}^* T_{2010} \\
&\quad + \gamma_{(t-1)2} P_{i(t-1)}{}^* T_{2008} + \gamma_{(t-1)3} P_{i(t-1)}{}^* T_{2009} + \gamma_{(t-1)4} P_{i(t-1)}{}^* T_{2010} \\
&\qquad + \gamma_{(t-2)3} P_{i(t-2)}{}^* T_{2009} + \gamma_{(t-2)4} P_{i(t-2)}{}^* T_{2010} \\
&\qquad\qquad + \gamma_{(t-3)4} P_{i(t-3)}{}^* T_{2010} \\
&+ X_{it} \beta_3 + \varepsilon_{it} \qquad\qquad\qquad\qquad\qquad\qquad\qquad \text{Equation (iii)}
\end{aligned}
$$

where D is the annualized difference between the outcome of interest in year t and baseline for employee i; α_i is employee fixed effect; P_{it}, $P_{i(t-1)}$, $P_{i(t-3)}$, and $P_{i(t-4)}$ are program participation in the current year, the prior year, two years ago, three years ago, and four years ago, respectively; T_{2007}, T_{2008}, T_{2009}, and T_{2010} are indicators of calendar years 2007 to 2010, respectively, with the reference year being 2005; X_{it} is a vector of time varying employee characteristics, and ε_{it} is the error term.

In the simulations, as illustrated in Table B4, E_t, E_{t-1}, E_{t-3}, and E_{t-4} are the effects of current participation on the outcomes in the current year, the following year, two years later, three years later, and four years later, respectively. So the participation in 2006 results in an effect of E_t in 2006, E_{t1} in 2007, E_{t2} in 2008, E_{t3} in 2009, and E_{t4} in 2010. By the same token, participation in 2007 results an effect of $E_t + \gamma_{t1}$ in 2007, $E_{t1} + \gamma_{(t-1)2}$ in 2008, $E_{t2} + \gamma_{(t-2)3}$ in 2009, and $E_{t3} + \gamma_{(t-3)4}$ in 2010. If an employee participates in the

Table B4: Simulated Cumulative Effects of Multiyear Program Participation

Participation Year	Outcome Year				
	2006	**2007**	**2008**	**2009**	**2010**
2006	E_t	E_{t1}	E_{t2}	E_{t3}	E_{t4}
2007	-	$E_t + \gamma_{t1}$	$E_{t1} + \gamma_{(t-1)2}$	$E_{t2} + \gamma_{(t-2)3}$	$E_{t3} + \gamma_{(t-3)4}$
2008	-	-	$E_t + \gamma_{t2}$	$E_{t1} + \gamma_{(t-1)3}$	$E_{t2} + \gamma_{(t-2)4}$
2009	-	-	-	$E_t + \gamma_{t3}$	$E_{t1} + \gamma_{(t-1)4}$
2010	-	-	-	-	$E_t + \gamma_{t4}$

program in all five years, we will observe in 2006 an effect of E_t (summation of the first column), (E_{t1} + $E_t + \gamma_{t1}$) in 2007 (summation of the second column), ($E_{t2} + E_{t1} + \gamma_{(t-1)2} + E_t + \gamma_{t2}$) in 2008 (summation of the third column), and so forth. The cumulative effect of participation in 2006 will be simply the summation of the first column; the cumulative effect of participation in 2006–2007 will be the summation of the first two columns; that of participation in 2006–2008 will be the summation of the first three columns; and so forth.

When the assumption that program effects differ across time does not hold, the calculation was simplified by removing the interaction effects between participation and calendar years. In effect, if an employee participates in the program in all five years, we will observe in 2006 an effect of E_t (summation of the first column), ($E_{t1} + E_t$) in 2007 (summation of the second column), ($E_{t2} + E_{t1} + E_t$) in 2008 (summation of the third column), and so forth. Again, the cumulative effect of participation in 2006–2007 will be the summation of the first two columns; that of participation in 2006–2010 will be the summation of all the five columns. Our analysis indicates that program participation shows differential effects over time only in regressions where BMI is the dependent variable. In the BMI regression, the differential effect appears statistically significant only for 2010. Given that we have limited sample size in 2010 (88 observations), we decided to use regression results without interaction terms between program participation and calendar years.

Multivariate Analysis for the Effect of Incentives

We use multivariate regression models to estimate the impact of incentives on measures of wellness program uptake, such as HRA completion rates, program participation rates, and changes in health status.

The regression models aim at addressing two challenges in estimating the effect of incentives on the outcomes of interest.

(1) There is a possibility that incentive-offering is endogenous to the outcomes of interest. For example, an employer may offer incentives for HRA completion, because the HRA completion rate is low. Similarly, an employer could decide to incentivize participation in a weight control program, if obesity rates are high.

(2) We do not observe factors that may change within an employer over time and confound our findings. For example, we do not observe the variability in how employers (or program vendors) implement the program. An employer may switch its program vendor, potentially changing program implementation, or may increase outreach efforts in later years. These program changes within an employer over time affect program participation or health status. Without controlling for program implementation characteristics, the effects of incentives would be either under- or overestimated.

To address (1), we used employer fixed effects, which allowed us to control for unobserved employer characteristics. These unobserved employer characteristics may affect incentive offering and outcomes of interest simultaneously. In some of the models, we used employee-level fixed effects, which absorbed the variation represented by employer fixed effects. Thus, employer indicators do not appear in some of the regression results. To address (2), we included in the regressions all possible interactions between employer indicators and calendar year indicators. These interaction terms would capture all the variation in program implementation that is not accounted for by the variation in incentives across employers and over time.

For HRA completion or lifestyle program participation, we tested simple logit models with employer fixed effects and robust standard errors, linear probability models with employee fixed effects, and logit models with employee fixed effects. Logit models with employee fixed effects automatically discarded a majority of the data because of no variation in the outcome within employees, whereas linear probability models may generate predicted probabilities that are greater than one or smaller than zero. Given that the results are similar across different models, we adopted the following simple logit model with robust standard errors:

$$\text{Logit}\,(p) = \beta_0 + C\beta_1 + E\beta_2 + T\beta_3 + (E*T)\,\beta_4 + X\beta_5 \qquad \text{Equation (iv)}$$

where p is the probability of HRA completion or lifestyle program participation, C represents incentive amount or incentive indicators, E is a vector of employer indicators, T is a vector of year indicators, E*T represents interaction terms between employer and year indicators, and X is a vector of employee characteristics. Employee characteristics include employee age, gender, enrollment in a capitated health plan, region, Charlson comorbidity index, prior year PMPM medical cost, prior year inpatient admissions, and prior year emergency department visits. The HRA completion regressions were performed for all employees in the final analytic sample using incentives for HRA completion only, and the program participation regressions were conducted using incentives for lifestyle program participation among those who were eligible for a program.

For smoking cessation, we used a similar approach to that for HRA completion as described above— Equation (iv)—except that we required that all employees be smokers in the baseline year. We considered total incentives–for both HRA completion and lifestyle program participation–as the exposure measure, because both HRA completion and lifestyle program participation may affect health behavior and health status.

For BMI, exercise, and total cholesterol, we examined difference-in-difference estimates of the effects of total incentives because, unlike smoking status, which is a dichotomous variable, these dependent variables are continuous variables. We tested whether incentive effectiveness varies across calendar years and region when appropriate. In health behavior and health status regressions, we did not include program participation, because it is on the causal path way between incentives and outcomes. The models take the following form:

$$D_{it} = \alpha_i + I_{it}\beta_1 + X_{it}\beta_2 + T\beta_3 + \varepsilon_{it} \qquad \text{Equation (v)}$$

where D is the annualized difference between the outcome of interest in year t and baseline for employee i, α_i is the employee fixed effect, I_{it} is a vector of total incentives, X_{it} is a vector of time varying employee characteristics, T is a vector of year indicators, and ε_{it} is the error term.

Limitations of the CCA data analysis

Several limitations remain in spite of our efforts to address the endogeneity between program participation and the outcomes of interest (health behavior, health outcomes, and medical costs), or between incentives offering and HRA completion, lifestyle program participation, health behaviors, and health outcomes. There might be some residual bias that we were not able to control for in the analysis.

- The CCA database contains a convenience sample of employers. In other words, it is not a representative sample of all employers in the United States. In addition, the sample includes only large employers with an employment size of 8,000 or more. Our results may not be generalizable to smaller employers or employers in other industries. It is quite possible that program participation effects differ in smaller employers compared to larger ones.

- Currently, the CCA database contains only a few employers, which limits the variation in employer-level characteristics, such as average employee income, industry, employment size, and incentives offered. In particular, the limited variation in incentives prevents us from reaching robust conclusions regarding the impact of incentives on lifestyle program participation, health behaviors, and health outcomes.

- Health behaviors and health outcome variables are from HRAs. These are likely self-reported data, although some employers do incorporate screening data into HRA, such as total cholesterol. Limitations of self-reported data certainly apply here.

- Given our relatively large sample of employees, several requirements in our analysis considerably reduce the sample size in the final analytic sample. First, the use of a difference-in-difference approach requires that all individuals have at least two years of data and that all program participants have one year of data before program participation (the baseline year data were used to match participants and nonparticipants). Second, we included employee years only when full 12 months of data were available, because linear extrapolation of partial year data could be potentially problematic. Third, we also excluded employee years if employees were enrolled in a capitated plan. Finally, program participation data and outcome data were required to conduct our analyses. This is particularly a problem for outcomes derived from HRA data, such as exercise, smoking status, BMI, and cholesterol.

- We were not able to control for time-variant characteristics that are not available in our data. For example, only lifestyle management program but not disease management program data are available in the CCA database. Lack of information on disease management program participation could bias our estimates.

- We were not able to fully control for differential motivation to change behavior or improve health when comparing participants to nonparticipants. This is particularly a concern for such health behaviors as exercise and smoking. Participants are typically better motivated to change health behavior and, therefore, we might have overestimated the program impacts. Since we include individual fixed effects in the models, the residual bias may come only from motivation that changes over time within the same individual. In other words, if motivation does not change over time within the same individual, differential motivation between participants and nonparticipants does not bias our estimates.

- Our analysis could not account for variation in program components, implementation, and outreach activities across the wellness programs offered by the employers in our analytic sample. In our analysis, we could examine only whether any program participation has an effect on our outcomes of interest—we were not able to examine the differential effects of various program features on outcomes. In addition, our analysis did not investigate dose-response effects of program intervention because of a lack of reliable data.

References

111th Congress (2010). Patient Protection and Affordable Care Act.

Aldana, S. G., R. M. Merrill, et al. (2005). "Financial impact of a comprehensive multisite workplace health promotion program." *Preventive Medicine* **40**(2): 131–137.

Baicker, K., D. Cutler, et al. (2010). "Workplace wellness programs can generate savings." *Health Affairs* **29**(2): 304–311.

Barham, K., S. West, et al. (2011). "Diabetes prevention and control in the workplace: a pilot project for county employees." *J Public Health Manag Pract* **17**(3): 233–241.

Cahill, K., M. Moher, et al. (2008). "Workplace interventions for smoking cessation." *Cochrane Database of Systematic Reviews* (4): CD003440.

Cahill, K., and R. Perera (2011). "Competitions and incentives for smoking cessation." *Cochrane Database of Systematic Reviews* (4): CD004307.

Campbell, M. K., I. Tessaro, et al. (2002). "Effects of a tailored health promotion program for female blue-collar workers: health works for women." *Preventive Medicine* **34**(3): 313–323.

Centers for Disease Control and Prevention (2010). "Chronic Disease Overview. 2011." As of March 11, 2013:
http://www.cdc.gov/chronicdisease/overview/index.htm

Centers for Disease Control and Prevention (2011). "How much physical activity do adults need?" As of March 11, 2013:
http://www.cdc.gov/physicalactivity/everyone/guidelines/adults.html

Cook, R. F., D. W. Billings, et al. (2007). "A field test of a web-based workplace health promotion program to improve dietary practices, reduce stress, and increase physical activity: randomized controlled trial." *Journal of Medical Internet Research* **9**(2): e17.

Darling, H., D. Dannel, et al. (2011). *Large Employers' 2012 Health Plan Design Changes.* Washington, D.C.: National Business Group on Health.
http://capsules.kaiserhealthnews.org/wp-content/uploads/2011/08/2012-NBGH-Plan-Design-Survey-Report-Embargoed-Edition.pdf

Davis, L. M., D. Golinelli, et al. (2008). *The National Computer Security Survey (NCSS) – Final Methodology.* Santa Monica, Calif.: RAND Corporation, TR–544. As of March 11, 2013:
http://www.rand.org/pubs/technical_reports/TR544.html

DeVol, R., A. Bedroussian, et al. (2007). *An Unhealthy America: The Economic Burden of Chronic Disease – Charting a New Course to Save Lives and Increase Productivity and Economic Growth.*

Faghri, P. D., E. Blozie, et al. (2008). "The role of tailored consultation following health-risk appraisals in employees' health behavior." *Journal of Occupational and Environmental Medicine/American College of Occupational and Environmental Medicine* **50**(12): 1378–1385.

Federal Register (2012). Incentives for Nondiscriminatory Wellness Programs in Group Health Plans. Washington, D.C. Proposed Rule: 77 Fed. Reg, 70620–70642

Federal Register (2013). Incentives for Nondiscriminatory Wellness Programs in Group Health Plans. Washington, D.C.: Final Rule: [Contemporanesouly published],

French, S. A., L. J. Harnack, et al. (2010). "Worksite environment intervention to prevent obesity among metropolitan transit workers." *Preventive Medicine* **50**(4): 180–185.

Galinsky, E., and K. Matos (2012). *2012 National Study of Employers.* New York: Families and Work Institute.
http://familiesandwork.org/site/research/reports/NSE_2012.pdf

Goetzel, R. Z., D. Shechter, et al. (2007). "Promising practices in employer health and productivity management efforts: findings from a benchmarking study." *Journal of Occupational and*

Environmental Medicine/American College of Occupational and Environmental Medicine **49**(2): 111–130.

Gold, D. B., D. R. Anderson, et al. (2000). "Impact of a telephone-based intervention on the reduction of health risks." *American Journal of Health Promotion* **15**(2): 97–106.

Healthy People 2020 (2011). "Healthy People 2020." As of March 11, 2013: http://www.healthypeople.gov/2020/about/default.aspx

Henke, R. M., R. Z. Goetzel, et al. (2011). "Recent experience in health promotion at Johnson & Johnson: lower health spending, strong return on investment." *Health Affairs* **30**(3): 490–499.

Herman, C. W., S. Musich, et al. (2006). "Effectiveness of an incentive-based online physical activity intervention on employee health status." *Journal of Occupational and Environmental Medicine/American College of Occupational and Environmental Medicine* **48**(9): 889–895.

Hewitt Associates (2010). *The Road Ahead: Under Construction with Increasing Tolls, Survey Findings.* Lincolnshire, Ill: Hewitt Associates, LLC. http://www.aon.com/attachments/thought-leadership/Hewitt_Survey_Findings_TheRoadAhead_2010.pdf

Hochart, C., and M. Lang (2011). "Impact of a comprehensive worksite wellness program on health risk, utilization, and health care costs." *Popul Health Manag* **14**(3): 111–116.

Hoffman, C., and K. Schwartz (2008). "Eroding access among nonelderly U.S. adults with chronic conditions: ten years of change." *Health Aff (Millwood)* **27**(5): w340–348.

Hoffman, H. (2012). "Oregon wellness program differs from other states." *Statesman Journal*

Hoovers: A Dun & Bradstreet Company (undated). "Website." As of March 7, 2013: http://subscriber.hoovers.com/H/home/index.html. Subscription required

Integrated Benefits Institute (2010). *IBI's Survey of HPM Practices (Presentation).*

James, J. (2012). "Health Policy Brief: Workplace Wellness Programs." *Health Affairs.*

KFF/HRET (2010). *Employer Health Benefits: 2010 Annual Survey.* Menlo Park, Calif; Chicago, Ill: Kaiser Family Foundation/Health Research and Educational Trust.

KFF/HRET (2011). *Employer Health Benefits: 2011 Annual Survey.* Menlo Park, Calif; Chicago, Ill.: Kaiser Family Foundation/Health Research and Educational Trust

KFF/HRET (2012). *Employer Health Benefits: 2012 Annual Survey.* Menlo Park, Calif; Chicago, Ill: Kaiser Family Foundation/Health Research and Educational Trust. http://ehbs.kff.org/pdf/2012/8345.pdf

Klautzer, L., S. Mattke, et al. (2012). "Can We Legally Pay People for Being Good? A Review of Current Federal and State Law on Wellness Program Incentives." *Inquiry Journal* **49**.

Kolbe-Alexander, T. L., K. I. Proper, et al. (2012). "Working on wellness (WOW): A worksite health promotion intervention programme." *BMC Public Health* **12**: 372.

Leeks, K. D., D. P. Hopkins, et al. (2010). "Worksite-based incentives and competitions to reduce tobacco use. A systematic review." *American Journal of Preventive Medicine* **38**(2 Suppl): S263–274.

Liu, H., K. M. Harris, et al. (2012). "Effect of an Employer-Sponsored Health and Wellness Program on Medical Cost and Utilization." *Popul Health Manag.*

MacKinnon, D. P., D. L. Elliot, et al. (2010). "Long-term effects of a worksite health promotion program for firefighters." *American Journal of Health Behavior* **34**(6): 695–706.

Madison, K. M., K. G. Volpp, et al. (2011). "The law, policy, and ethics of employers' use of financial incentives to improve health." *J Law Med Ethics* **39**(3): 450–468.

Mastroianni, P. (2009). "ADA: Disability-Related Inquiries and Medical Examinations; Health Risk Assessment." As of March 11, 2013: http://www.eeoc.gov/eeoc/foia/letters/2009/ada_disability_medexam_healthrisk.html

Mattke, S., C. Schnyer, et al. (2012). "A Review of the US Workplace Wellness Market."

Mello, M. M., and M. B. Rosenthal (2008). "Wellness programs and lifestyle discrimination–the legal limits." *The New England Journal of Medicine* **359**(2): 192–199.

Mercer (2010). *National Survey of Employer-Sponsored Health Plans: 2009 Survey Report*. New York.

Mercer (2011). "Employers accelerate efforts to bring health benefit costs under control."   As:

Milani, R. V., and C. J. Lavie (2009). "Impact of worksite wellness intervention on cardiac risk factors and one-year health care costs." *The American Journal of Cardiology* **104**(10): 1389–1392.

NAICS (2011). "2007 North American Industry Classification System."   As of November 11, 2010: http://www.census.gov/cgi-bin/sssd/naics/naicsrch?chart=2007

National Business Group on Health (2010). *The Employee Mindset: Views, Behaviors and Solutions*. Lincolnshire, Ill; Washington, D.C.: Hewitt Associates.

National Center for Health Statistics (2012). *National Health Interview Survey, 2011 (machine-readable file and documentation)*. Hyattsville, Md. http://www.cdc.gov/nchs/nhis.htm.

Naydeck, B. L., J. A. Pearson, et al. (2008). "The impact of the highmark employee wellness programs on 4-year healthcare costs." *Journal of Occupational and Environmental Medicine/American College of Occupational and Environmental Medicine* **50**(2): 146–156.

Nichols, J. F., E. Wellman, et al. (2000). "Impact of a worksite behavioral skills intervention." *American Journal of Health Promotion* **14**(4): 218–221.

Nyce, S. (2010). *Boosting Wellness Participation Without Breaking the Bank*: Towers Watson. http://www.towerswatson.com/assets/pdf/2395/2395.pdf

Nyman, J. A., N. A. Barleen, et al. (2010). "The effectiveness of health promotion at the University of Minnesota: expenditures, absenteeism, and participation in specific programs." *Journal of Occupational and Environmental Medicine/American College of Occupational and Environmental Medicine* **52**(3): 269–280.

Osilla, K. C., K. Van Busum, et al. (2012). "Systematic review of the impact of worksite wellness programs." *The American Journal of Managed Care* **18**(2): e68–81.

Ozminkowski, R. J., R. Z. Goetzel, et al. (2000). "The impact of the Citibank, NA, health management program on changes in employee health risks over time." *Journal of Occupational and Environmental Medicine/American College of Occupational and Environmental Medicine* **42**(5): 502–511.

Pollard, T. (2008). "Western Diseases: An Evolutionary Perspective", Cambridge University Press.

PricewaterhouseCoopers (2010). *Health and Well-being Touchstone Survey, Executive Summary*. http://www.pwc.com/us/en/hr-management/publications/health-wellness-touchstone-survey-2012.jhtml

PricewaterhouseCoopers (2010). *The Price of Excess: Identifying Waste in Healthcare Spending*: Health Research Institute. http://www.pwc.com/us/en/healthcare/publications/the-price-of-excess.jhtml

Purath, J., A. M. Miller, et al. (2004). "A brief intervention to increase physical activity in sedentary working women." *The Canadian Journal of Nursing Research/Revue Canadienne de Recherche en Sciences Infirmieres* **36**(1): 76–91.

Racette, S. B., S. S. Deusinger, et al. (2009). "Worksite Opportunities for Wellness (WOW): effects on cardiovascular disease risk factors after 1 year." *Preventive Medicine* **49**(2–3): 108–114.

Schmidt, H. (2012). "Wellness incentives, equity, and the 5 groups problem." *American Journal of Public Health* **102**(1): 49–54.

Siegel, J. M., M. L. Prelip, et al. (2010). "A worksite obesity intervention: results from a group-randomized trial." *American Journal of Public Health* **100**(2): 327–333.

137

Terry, P. E., J. B. Fowles, et al. (2011). "The ACTIVATE study: results from a group-randomized controlled trial comparing a traditional worksite health promotion program with an activated consumer program." *Am J Health Promot* **26**(2): e64–73.

Tu, H., and R. Mayrell (2010). *Employer Wellness Initiatives Grow, but Effectiveness Varies Widely*: National Institute for Health Care Reform.

U.S. Department of Health and Human Services (2004). *Prevention: a Blueprint for Action. Appendix F– Incentives for Healthy Behavior*. Washington, DC. As of July 28, 2011: http://www.health.state.mn.us/divs/hpsc/hep/transform/resourcebook/preventiontab18.pdf

U.S. Department of Labor. "FAQs about the HIPAA Nondiscrimination Requirements."   As of April 6, 2011: http://www.dol.gov/ebsa/faqs/faq_hipaa_ND.html

Volpp, K. G. (2009). "Paying people to lose weight and stop smoking." *LDI Issue Brief* **14**(3): 1–4.

Volpp, K. G., D. A. Asch, et al. (2011). "Redesigning employee health incentives–lessons from behavioral economics." *N Engl J Med* **365**(5): 388–390.

Volpp, K. G., A. B. Troxel, et al. (2009). "A randomized, controlled trial of financial incentives for smoking cessation." *The New England Journal of Medicine* **360**(7): 699–709.